Traditional Herbal Remedies

&

Healing Herbal Teas

The Practical Beginner's Guide to Prepare at Home Your Own Natural Remedies with Medicinal Plants & Herbs

Natural Apothecary

Table of Content

Introduction

The use of plants for therapeutic and medicinal purposes has very ancient origins. Almost as old as man himself, in fact, it is believed that as early as prehistoric times man began to treat himself with plants. It is a fairly widespread theory that it was through observation and direct experience that man discovered that trees and plants held healing properties within themselves. Just as all knowledge and forms of knowledge arise from a need, healing with natural methods also followed this course. Primitive man had to survive in an environment deeply hostile to him, but that same environment also held the key to his survival.

By observing the world around him he understood which plants could be poisonous, which could provide nourishment, and which could heal wounds and relieve pain. This rudimentary knowledge of the healing properties of plants, combined with early experimentation and practice, led to the association of plants, berries, flowers, or trees with certain painful states or diseases.

As the human race evolved, this knowledge of the healing powers of plants began to be passed down from generation to generation, at first only orally, then also in writing, giving rise to the first figures of healers. The oldest written records date back to 3000 BC. This is a herbarium written in China that contained more than 200 uses of herbs for healing purposes. In 1500 BC in Luxor, Egypt, a papyrus was compiled containing the healing properties of more than 500 plants.

Unfortunately, during the Middle Ages herbal healing came to be associated with magic and witchcraft and found considerable difficulty in application. People avoided applying it lest they be accused of practicing magical arts. We have monks to thank for the fact that knowledge of herbal healing has come down to us; in fact, they took care to transcribe the most important materials from the various traditions so that they would not be lost.

This was around the year 1000 AD. At that time monks also began to care for the sick using the knowledge that came from the texts they transcribed. In the beginning, they went to the woods and fields to collect buds, berries, barks, flowers, shoots, herbs, and roots. Over time, however, they began to grow in their own gardens what they needed to cure and with which they created rich storehouses of medicinal herbs, supplies with which they could cure those in need.

The discovery of America marked an important milestone in herbal healing for two reasons. First, there was access to a new and considerable amount of plant varieties, and second, Native Americans were great connoisseurs of the healing powers of the herbs of their territories.

The Industrial Revolution marked a change in healing methods for humans, causing them to lose the traditional use of plants and herbs. With the move away from the countryside and great new technological breakthroughs, medicine also began to evolve, arriving today with great discoveries that have exponentially improved our life expectancy.

Just today, thanks to these great discoveries, we have begun to understand that combining the properties of plants, flowers, herbs, and trees with traditional medicine can give important benefits to our bodies, our health, and our well-being.

The events of the past two years have shown us how important and fragile our health can be, so it is important to preserve it and take care of it in the best way possible.

In the next few chapters, I will show you how the plants of the world around can help you feel better day after day. You will find out how to create your own plant reserve from scratch, what are the best ways to consume a plant based on the result you want to achieve, when and which part of each plant to harvest, and what are the uses of the various medicinal plants, and then I will share with you lots of recipes for herbal teas and plant-based remedies illustrating what they are useful for. In this way, you will be able to take advantage of the properties of plants simply and practically, on your own, and right at home.

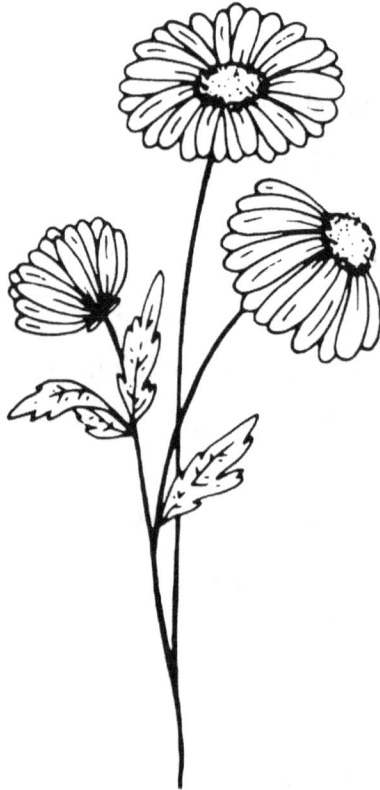

Chamomile

How to Exploit the Properties of Herbs and Plants

The main and most common method of harnessing the properties of plants at home is herbal tea. Herbal tea is, basically, an aqueous solution in which the medicinal principles of plants are diluted.

Water is the best and most important natural "solvent" for keeping the healing elements of herbs active, but for this to happen the quality of the water must be very high. The water must be as pure as possible because, in case of impurities or excessive limestone, the quality of the plant's healing principles would be affected.

When preparing herbal tea, it is very important not to use metal or enameled pots, because they would compromise the quality of the result.

Over-heating or re-heating herbal teas also compromises the quality of their healing properties. Since it is okay to drink or use them both cold and hot, my suggestion is to prepare the herbal tea just before consuming or using it if you need it hot. If, on the other hand, you need it cold, you can prepare the daily needed amount, store it in a glass pitcher, and sip it or use it when you need to.

It would be ideal to consume the herbal tea without the addition of sweeteners. If it is really impossible for you, however, absolutely avoid sugar or chemical sweeteners. The best option is honey, which goes wonderfully with all kinds of herbs.

Licorice is also an excellent option for sweetening your herbal teas, or at any rate to cover bitterness or too intense flavors. You can use licorice juice, an extract, or, more simply, add the chopped root to your herbal tea. If, on the other hand, it is the smell that you don't like and that makes it difficult to consume your herbal tea, there are numerous options available to you. The key is to keep in mind the properties and uses of what you are going to add to your herbal tea to make it more pleasant. To make it smell more pleasant you can use fresh or dried citrus peels, mint, green anise, vanilla, cinnamon, or cloves, just to name a few. Some aromatic herbs are also very useful for this purpose, for example, sage, thyme, and rosemary.

Herbal teas, to be most effective, should be consumed at certain times and under certain conditions according to their purpose and function:

Time	Mode	Function
Early morning	Empty stomach	Depurative, diuretic, and laxative
Mid-morning		Tonic for the heart, against coughs, antiseptic, and against rheumatism
Mid-afternoon		Tonic for the heart, against coughs, antiseptic, and against rheumatism
Before meals	30 minute before	anti-acidic and restorative
After meals		Digestive
Evening	Just before going to sleep	Relaxing, laxative, circulation-boosting, and sleep-aiding

You may have noticed that until now I have only ever used the term herbal tea, whereas you may have often heard of infusions, decoctions, and other names.

Herbal teas can be prepared in five ways, which are:

1. _Infusions_

2. _Decoctions_

3. _Macerates_

4. _Baths_

5. *Compresses*

We will now look in detail at each of these types of herbal teas, how to prepare them, how to use them, and why. Not all of them are to be drunk. We will analyze each kind individually, so in the remedies section, you will have a clear idea of the use, even if it will be well described in each remedy covered.

The basic concept is that plants and flowers should never be over-boiled because otherwise, they would lose their properties; whereas, on the other hand, the barks and roots, need a more extensive process to extract their active ingredients, so they need to be brought to a boil of a certain length to make a decoction.

1. Infusions

Infusion is prepared in a way similar to tea. Water is heated until just before it comes to a boil, poured over the herbs, leaving them to steep for 5 or 10 minutes, depending on the herbs used, and finally strained and then drunk.

This type of herbal tea is used for herbs, flowers, and more delicate plants whose principles would be lost due to water and excessive heat. For this reason, the water should never reach boiling point, otherwise, the active ingredients of the infused plants would be lost. If you accidentally heat the water too much, let it sit for a few minutes before pouring it over the herbs.

The infusion is usually prepared once a day and then consumed at appropriate times throughout the day. As I mentioned earlier, herbal teas should not be re-heated, so you can store the excess in a glass thermos flask, or consume it cold throughout the day. Both are good alternatives that also help you consume your infusion according to seasonality. There might be some exceptions, so follow the guidelines specified in each remedy description.

Let's see how to prepare your infusion. This is a basic guideline, in fact, the ratio between the quantity of water and the number of herbs will vary according to the use of the infusion. For example, an infusion prepared to relieve an inconvenience will need a higher quantity of plants than one prepared to just have a pleasant and healthy drink during your day. The amount to be used is also often influenced by the type of plant being used, but the one below is a good general outline to stick to.

Ingredients:

- 2 cups of water

- 1.24 oz of dried herb

Or

- 2.82 oz of fresh herb

Tools needed:

- A glass, ceramic, or earthenware teapot with a lid

- A strainer

- A glass pitcher or glass thermos flask

- A drinking cup

Preparation method:

1. Bring the water as close to boiling point as possible without reaching it.

2. Meanwhile, place the herb in the bottom of the teapot and then pour the water over it as soon as it has reached the desired temperature.

3. Close the lid of the teapot and let it steep for a maximum of 10-15 minutes (the minimum time is 3 to 5 minutes, but it will depend on the herb used). I recommend using a timer for optimal success of your brew, especially until you get the hang of it or if you tend to get distracted and risk letting it steep for hours.

4. After the given time has elapsed, place the strainer on the pitcher to store the brew or on the thermos and strain it.

5. Sweeten it with a drizzle of honey, if you like.

6. Drink your first warm cup, make sure it's not too hot, cause you don't want to get burned.

You do not necessarily have to consume the infusion during the whole day. You can also consume it in a much smaller space of time that suits you if the remedy allows it. Keep in mind that, in general, the infusion gives its best when drunk as soon as it is made, but you can safely keep it for several hours as long as you use a suitable container, and as I have already advised glass is perfect for this purpose. If you store the pitcher in the refrigerator, most infusions will keep for up to 24 hours. The suggestion is to brew your infusion daily. Personally, I brew a pitcher of infusion every day in the summer and keep it stored in the refrigerator to drink it nice and fresh the next day, as a healthy alternative to the chemical and sugary drinks commonly used to quench one's thirst. The active ingredients might be a tad less strong with this method, but the solution is infinitely healthier than most of the sodas we end up consuming in the summer to seek relief from the heat.

Here are some examples of herbs suitable for infusion:

- Chamomile

- Mallow

- Lemon balm

- Elderberry

- Orange blossom

- Aromatic herbs (Laurel, Sage, Oregano, Fennel)

- Calendula

- Linden

There are also some roots that, if harvested tender enough, can be consumed by infusion:

- Valerian

- Gentian

- Rhubarb

2. Decoctions

A decoction is prepared by adding cold water to the herbs and simmering it for no longer than 20 minutes. Decoction takes a little longer to prepare than infusion, so it would be easier for you to prepare all the daily quantity at one time and preserve it throughout the day.

This form of herbal tea is used for roots (especially hard ones), seeds, some types of berries, and woody, twiggy herbs. Basically, a decoction is used to extract the active ingredients from the hard parts of plants.

Here's how to prepare your daily portion of decoction, keeping in mind that the same applies to the herb-to-water ratio as for infusions:

Ingredients:

- 3 cups of water (water reduces during boiling)

- 1.24 oz of dried herb

Or

- 2.3 oz of fresh herb

Tools needed:

- Pot (not enameled, nor bare metal), for preparation

- Colander

- Glass jug with lid, glass thermos flask, or ceramic teapot with lid, for the daily storage

Preparation method:

1. Place the herb in the bottom of the pot and pour cold water over it.

2. Place the pot on the stove and bring the water to a boil.

3. Let your decoction boil for no more than 20 minutes (each remedy described further on will have the exact boiling time). During this time the water should lose part of its volume, usually, 3 cups become about 2 cups, after boiling and filtering.

4. Turn off the stove and let it steep for an additional 10 minutes (not all remedies need this extra stepping time, again each remedy described will have detailed timed instructions), then strain it by placing the strainer over the pitcher or teapot and pouring out the decoction.

5. Sweeten the decoction with a little honey, if you like.

6. Drink your first warm cup, make sure it's not too hot, cause you don't want to get burned.

Decoctions are very similar to infusions in terms of consumption. They should be consumed hot or lukewarm, but not boiling. It is also fine to drink them at room temperature. The preparation should not be re-heated so as not to lose its properties. It can last several hours in the storage jug and up to 24 hours if kept cool.

Consuming infusions and decoctions very cold is not exactly ideal, because they lose a small part of their active ingredients. However, as I explained in the section on infusions, consuming them cold in the summer is a healthy alternative to summer drinks, so it is better to lose a small portion of active ingredients than to consume sugary, unhealthy commercial drinks.

Decoctions, like infusions, can also be used to make washes in certain areas of the body or to wet gauze to apply to the skin.

Here are some examples of herbs suitable for decoctions:

- Hawthorn fruits

- Horsetail

- Mallow leaves

- Nettle leaves

- Artichoke leaves

- Willow bark

- Horse chestnut bark

- Licorice root

- Echinacea

- Rhubarb

You will notice that rhubarb root was also mentioned in infusions. Numerous plants can be used in both ways, that is, prepared as an infusion and as a decoction. However, the results produced on the body by the same plant will be very different depending on its preparation. For example, rhubarb infusion is an excellent digestive, while decoction helps liver regularity and acts as a laxative. Horsetail infusion helps diuresis, while decoction helps the body replenish mineral salts.

3. Macerates

The macerate is prepared by immersing the plant, properly shredded, in water at room temperature, where it must macerate for a time ranging from a few hours to a few days.

This solution is used for all those plants that have active ingredients that can be released in water but are too sensitive to heat. This method is used to avoid losing the properties altogether.

The key element for good steeping is accuracy in chopping the herbs. If they are chopped too coarsely, a good macerate will not be obtained. Conversely, if the herbs are meticulously chopped up, a macerate rich in active ingredients will be obtained.

Given the longer preparation time, a slightly higher than daily amount can be prepared, although daily preparation remains ideal, at least for those that require only a few hours of maceration.

It is imperative that the macerate rest in a well-covered container that is not exposed to direct light. Before consumption, it should be carefully filtered like the decoction and infusion. It is very useful for extracting the properties of those plants that are too sensitive to heat, which we would otherwise have no way of using, although, unfortunately, it is much less practical to prepare than infusions and decoctions. The same considerations made in the previous sections also apply here for ingredient ratios.

Ingredients:

- 2 cups of water or alcohol

- 2.3 oz of finely and carefully chopped fresh herb

Or

- 1.24 oz of dried herb

Tools needed:

- A glass, ceramic or earthenware teapot, or container with a lid

- A strainer

- A glass pitcher with a lid for storage

- A drinking cup

Preparation method:

1. Very finely chop the fresh herb chosen for the macerate and place it in the teapot or steeping container.

2. Pour cold water or alcohol (depending on the instructions of the remedy) directly over the chopped herb, put the lid on, and let it macerate away from direct sunlight.

3. Steep for anywhere from a few hours to a few days, depending on the macerate you need to prepare.

4. When it is time, strain through a strainer and pour the macerate into the storage jug.

5. Sweeten with a drizzle of honey, if you like.

6. Drink according to the instructions of the remedy.

Here are some examples of herbs suitable for macerates:

Bearberry makes an antiseptic macerate and is particularly useful against cystitis.

Althea protects the intestines and helps them perform their functions properly and is particularly useful against gastritis.

Bearberry can also be used in infusion, but it yields a much less effective compound than that obtained from the macerate.

4. Baths

Baths, also called "full baths" by some, are immersions of the entire body in hot water with the addition of the desired herbs. It is a bit like taking a bath in a large cup of infusion.

The difference between a "full bath" and a so-called "sitz bath" lies in the amount of the body that is immersed. The full bath involves soaking up to the chest, while the "sitz bath" involves soaking only up to the lower back, say up to the kidneys. It is also possible to take partial baths where only the desired part is immersed.

In baths, one then immerses the body, or a part of it, in a solution of water in which an infusion or decoction is diluted, for a maximum time of 20 to 30 minutes. The amount of herbs needed for the infusion varies according to the type of bath. For a "sitz bath", half the amount needed for a full bath will be used, while for a local soak even less. (You will get precise instructions on each remedy in the specific chapter).

5. Compresses

Compresses are also called poultices. They involve applying a decoction of herbs directly to the part to be treated and using a bandage to wrap the herbs. Sometimes, you might have to soak a gauze or a cotton cloth onto an infusion, and apply that directly to the area to treat.

The poultice must have a thick, pasty consistency so that it can be spread on the desired area and then covered in bandages. To make it, a good amount of dried herbs must be cooked in water. Alternatively, fresh herbs can be pounded directly with a mortar.

The mixture should always be applied lukewarm or cold, never too hot because it may damage the area to which it is applied.

Herbal teas, in the three drinkable forms of infusion, decoction, and macerate, are extremely useful for:

- Aiding digestion

- Improving the quality of sleep

- Regularizing the bowels

- Sedate coughs and colds

- Calming anxiety and agitation

- Promote diuresis

Very often they are also associated with drug therapies for chronic diseases to give additional support.

Let's say that, in general, herbal teas help relieve discomforts of various degrees and, in many cases, prevent them.

We will see in the remedies section many specific uses of herbal teas, derived from the active ingredients of the herbs used in the preparation of each remedy. Depending on the plants used, their combination, and the type of preparation, different results will be obtained.

To avoid undesirable reactions of the body, it is recommended never to exceed 5 different herbs in the same herbal tea; in addition, an herbal tea should never contain caffeine. This is why, in this book, I haven't mentioned tea leaves.

The composition of a herbal tea should follow the pattern shown below:

1. *The basic remedy*: One or more herbs with specific active ingredients for the desired treatment.

2. *The adjuvant*: One or more herbs that can help the basic remedy to be more effective.

3. *The compliment*: One or more herbs that can impart a more pleasant taste.

4. *The corrector*: One or more herbs that can improve characteristics such as color, smell, palate sensation, ...

An herbal tea, therefore, should contain a maximum of 5 herbs appropriate to this composition scheme. The most popular herbal teas are those detoxifying, depurative or draining, calming or relaxing, fat-burning or slimming; however, in the remedies section, I will share with you a much wider range of uses, for all the little discomforts you may encounter in daily life.

How to Source the Best Ingredients

The quality of ingredients in herbal teas is crucial to ensure good results. By good quality I mean, first and foremost, that the herbs should be grown only with natural fertilizers and be completely organic and not treated in any way with pesticides and chemical fertilizers.

The herbs must, in addition, be dried properly and always stored optimally, to preserve intact the active ingredients that we are going to extract for consumption with the herbal tea.

The options available to you are not much, really only two. You can find a trusted herbalist shop that can get you products of the quality you need, or you can get the herbs and plants you need yourself by organizing a greenhouse, a garden, and gathering in nature what you need and cannot produce. The second option is, of course, the best. It allows you to have the highest quality plants, herbs, flowers, and also gives you access to fresh herbs at different times of the year, an advantage not to be underestimated at all. On the other hand, it is a choice not suitable for everyone for a variety of reasons. You need space, for example, a garden, a small plot of land, or at least a nice balcony. It takes time to take care of the plants as they grow, and finally, it takes time to process them, and prepare them for storage for the long months of use.

Since this is the best method, I would like to go through all the important steps from harvesting to final storage so that you know them and know their importance, even if you should decide to opt to buy them.

Also, knowing these steps could be useful, because you might get lucky and discover someone with a wonderful botanical garden and a nice greenhouse, who might allow you to harvest your plants in his or her garden. This would allow you to have first-rate herbs while avoiding the difficult and labor-intensive part of growing them.

The herbs and plants that you will consume fresh in your herbal teas will be subject only to the harvesting stage, except in the case of the macerate where they will also have to be crushed properly.

The herbs and plants that you will dry, on the other hand, will go through a 4-step process:

1. *Harvesting*

2. *Drying*

3. *Storing*

4. *Crushing*

Let's analyze each stage in detail.

1. Harvesting

To get the best out of your herbal teas, you will need to harvest your herbs at the time when they contain the highest amount of active ingredients. Since this is a topic of high importance you will find a harvesting scheme in the next chapter, where you will find what part of the plant to harvest in what season. Harvesting periods, in fact, vary according to the part of the plant you want to use.

As anticipated in the introduction to this chapter, the quality of the plants you are going to harvest is critical, so unless they come from your own botanical garden, you should be very careful about where you harvest them.

Do not harvest your plants in dirty or polluted places where the plants may have come in contact with pesticides, heavy metals, or other toxic substances, perhaps dumped by some nearby factory.

Never collect your plants at the side of a road, no matter how much traffic is on it.

When harvesting parts of trees or plants that have a long life, keep in mind that the older the plant, the more active ingredients it will have. Determining the number of active ingredients present, however, is not only the age of the plant. Other determining factors are climate, temperature, and light. Other determining factors are the altitude at which the plant grows, the latitude, and the type of soil. All of these determine the chemical reactions of the plant, accentuating some characteristics over others. For example, altitude determines and conditions the amount of essential oil produced by the plant, while soil determines the quality of the plant and the speed at which it grows.

Let us now look at the best way and time to harvest the various parts of the plants.

Woody stems and barks

Woody stems should be harvested in winter. They Should be harvested before buds begin to sprout.

The bark should be collected in winter, before budding, if the tree is an adult. If the tree is still young, the best time to harvest is in fall. Exceptions are resinous plants and also conifers, whose bark should be collected in spring because that is when the sap rises.

Flowers

They should be collected in bud or, at any rate, long before the bloom reaches its apex.

Those that are to be collected during their bloom should be collected together with some leaves. Those to be harvested in bud are mainly herbs, for example, thyme, oregano, sage, and mint. If they are still in bud, the pollen will be jealously guarded inside. Once the flower has hatched, bees and insects will have carried away the pollen and nectar, depriving the flower of some of its active ingredients.

Plants

Whole plants should be harvested at the time of their full development. Some plants require a 2-year cycle to reach this full development, in which case they can be harvested only in their second year.

Fruits

Fruits should be picked ripe, at the peak of ripening, and when they have already taken on their beautiful color.

Seeds

Those inside the fruit should be harvested when the fruit is ripe.

Those on the plants, on the other hand, should be harvested before the plant loses them on its own, so before they begin to dry. Seeds should not be harvested on rainy or wet days, only on days when the weather is nice and dry. They should also always be harvested at times of day when the dew has already evaporated. Dusk is a good time and so is morning, if you wait precisely until the dew has left the plant.

Leaves and stems

Leaves should be harvested before flowering because they are still young. You should always harvest the topmost leaves. The lowest leaves are born first and are, therefore, the most wasted and deteriorated. There are a few exceptions, for example, Belladonna, whose leaves should be harvested only after the plant has flowered. The stems should also be harvested at the same time as is most suitable for the leaves, i.e., before flowering, when they are still very young.

Buds

Shoots on the plants should be harvested when the bud is still completely closed and protected inside the dark, stiff leaflet that surrounds it.

Bulbs

They should be harvested at the end of the flowering stage when the wilted petals begin to detach from the flower corolla.

Tubers

They should be harvested at the time of flowering.

Roots

Roots should be harvested in spring if the plant from which they are collected is a perennial plant. They should, on the other hand, be harvested in the fall if it is an annual plant. This is because they should be harvested at the plant's dormant stage.

2. Drying

Once we have harvested what we are interested in, we need to proceed to dry it. Drying must be carried out immediately after harvesting. With this process, you are going to remove most of the water present in the plant.

As soon as you have harvested the plants you are interested in you must, first of all, clean them. They may be muddy or even just dusty. You will have to wash them thoroughly, but gently so as not to damage them, and then you will have to dry them with hot air.

Special care should be taken to wash the roots, which are usually particularly dirty and full of soil. They should be washed very well to remove any residue, and then they should be pat-dried. Before they can be dried for storing, they should be cut into 1 to 2 cm pieces for two reasons. First, larger pieces would take too long to dry properly. Second, once dried it would be too difficult to cut them into pieces of appropriate size for use, so it is much more useful and practical to do it before.

Let's look at the drying steps together. The first step is to put your plants in the open air, exposed directly to the sun until they begin to wilt. You will need to divide the various plants, but also the various parts of each plant.

The second step, however, can be done in two ways. The easiest and quickest method is to use an oven or an electric dryer, but it can prove to be an expensive option because it takes quite a long time and you have to leave the appliances on and running. In addition, if the drying process is carried out in the summer, prolonged use of the oven in the house can be unpleasant.

Despite the energy and heat factor, it remains the quickest and most practical method. You simply have to put the plant parts divided by plant type and by plant part into the oven (or dryer). Plant parts that are exposed to the air should be dried at a temperature of 95°F (not to be exceeded), we are talking about leaves, flowers, stems, and so on. The parts of the plant that do not live exposed to air, such as the roots, should be dried at 122°F, you can go up to a maximum of 140°F, but you cannot exceed this temperature. The average time for drying with this method is between 12 and 24 hours, depending on the amount of water contained in the parts you are going to dry.

As an alternative to an oven or an electrical dryer, you can finish the drying process naturally, in a dry ventilated room positioned always in the shade, such as an attic, a loft, or a basement.

If the room you plan to use has windows you will need to screen them to create shade and prevent sunlight from penetrating. You will, however, have to make sure that air continues to circulate freely to allow the drying process to take place properly. Burlap sheets are very useful for this purpose, because their weave is sufficient to shield light, but allow air to circulate and penetrate through the window on which they are placed.

Once you have prepared the room you will need to separate the various parts of the various plants and then prepare them for drying.

Plants, stems and small woody stems: You can make small bundles loosely tied, do not tie them too tightly and hang them upside down. To do this, you will either have to place special hooks to the ceiling or set up a bar, again attached to the ceiling and tie the bundles to the bar. Alternatively, you can arrange your plants on special trellises. These are small frames to which a net is attached, allowing air to pass through and water to leave the plant. You will have to spread your plants and stems on these drying racks, making sure that no layer thicker than 1 inch is created, otherwise they will not dry properly. Every day you will have to take care of turning them over so that you do not run the risk of them fermenting and spoiling before you have completed your drying operation. Usually, it will take 15 to 20 days for complete drying, but of course, the time depends on the amount of water contained in the plants you are drying.

Flowers, roots, and leaves: You will simply deposit them in the bottom of a small box in a layer of no more than 1 inch, remembering to keep them separated from each other by plant and type. Then you will need to cover each box with a very heavy cotton cloth or burlap. The purpose is always to block light and allow air to pass through. The roots need about 15 to 20 days to dry. The leaves, on the other hand, need one week to 10 days. The flowers, finally, only 3 or 4 days. Again, the times are relative to the amount of water contained, but let's say they are fairly accurate arbitrary times.

Berries: You can lay them in a single layer on the bottom of a very low-sided carton. Drying time is around 2 to 3 weeks.

Seeds: Seeds require 2 stages of drying. You will first need to dry the pod or umbrella in which they are contained and it will take about a week. You do this by leaving them lying in a thin layer on a trellis. Once the pod or umbrella is dried, you will have to pass them through your hands to crush them. You will have to do this in a sieve so that the seeds are separated from the waste. Once you have cleaned the seeds from the useless parts, you will have to let them dry for another 7 days.

Proper drying is of paramount importance to ensure the quality and longevity of the herbs you are preparing for your herbal teas. If herbs and plants are dried and stored incorrectly they can develop toxins that are, indeed, toxic to the body. Therefore, not only would your herbal tea lose all of its active ingredients, but even risk becoming harmful.

Establishing proper drying, fortunately, is quite simple: you will have to pass the plant through your hands. If what you are touching feels dry to the touch and does not leave you with any kind of residue or trace of moisture, then your herbs are dry to the right degree.

There is also a little trick that you can use when you are just starting out or whenever you are in doubt. You will need an airtight jar, inside of which you should put a few small pieces of what you are drying. Close the jar tightly and let it sit for a few days. If droplets will form on the walls of the jar, it means that your plant has not yet lost all its moisture and needs to dry out some more. If, on the other hand, no moisture droplets appear on the walls of the jar, then your plant is dry enough and you can proceed to the next step.

3. Storing

As we said in the previous chapter, drying and storing must be approached with care and caution to avoid the deterioration of the plants you want to preserve.

A proper drying process, such as the one described in the previous section, is the key element for proper preservation. In fact, removing water prevents the major causes of deterioration.

Spoilage is usually caused by mold, bacteria, or pests such as moths, butterflies, and cockroaches. Dehydration prevents mold and bacteria from proliferating, preventing these two causes of spoilage from affecting our herbs and plants. Avoiding pests, on the other hand, requires only a few simple actions aimed at ensuring good quality storage.

Herbs must necessarily be stored in the dark, so in containers where no light gets through and, above all, tightly closed. Tin cans are ideal. Terracotta jars, or ceramic ones, like those in old pharmacies, for instance, do very well. The option that I find most practical and space-saving is to use paper bags. You need ones that are a bit dark and made of very thick and heavy paper, like the ones used at the grocery store. After filling the bag with your herbs and plants, you will need to seal it tightly and carefully with tape.

Whichever storage option you choose, remember to mark on the package the name of the plant, the part stored, the date of harvest, and the date of storage. This will help you always know the contents of your stash and how long you have been storing that product.

Keep in mind that the longer you store your herbs and plants, the weaker the active ingredient in them will become until it disappears. The advice is, therefore, to renew your stash every year, which is an adequate storage time to keep the active ingredients alive. This means that you should not store excessive amounts of herbs. At first, it will be difficult to estimate how much you may actually need in a year, but with time you will become proficient in this as well.

The storing phase is also very important even if you buy your herbs from a trusted herbalist or from monasteries (another place where you can find a wide selection of high-quality herbs). First, it would be ideal to make sure that the herbalist in the first place does not sell you herbs that are too old and have lost much of their active ingredients. Then, you should buy small quantities of herbs and replace them only after you run out. The concepts of storage also remain the same for the herbs you buy. You need closed containers through which no light will pass, such as tin jars, terracotta jars, ceramic jars with lids, or dark, heavy paper bags tape-closed. Again, I would use labels with the name of the plant, the part contained in that particular container, the date of purchase, and, if the herbalist can provide it, the date of drying. These are useful tricks to get the highest quality in your herbal teas, whether the herbs are your own or you buy them.

4. Crushing

When you prepare an herbal tea, to make sure that the active ingredients in the plant can be quickly extracted from the water, you must have the herb or plant crushed into small pieces. Please note, I said "small pieces," I did not say "pulverized."

Once a week, you must take enough plants from your stash to cover the entire week. You must carefully store the leftover and prepare to crush the quantity you will consume later in the week. Once crushed, the herb quickly loses its active ingredients, which last, precisely, about a week. That is why you will have to do this weekly and cannot do it for your entire supply after drying and before storage.

The ideal tool for crushing is the stone mortar, being very careful to break the plants into small pieces, without pulverizing them.

I do not recommend wooden mortars because they are difficult to clean and always remain somewhat impregnated with the other elements you previously pound in that same mortar. There are some metal versions, however, which are likely to release harmful elements into your herbs. For the same reason, I advise against using kitchen blenders or food grinders. The metal blades could release elements into your herbs, plus, because of their power, you would risk pulverizing the herbs instead of getting the small chunks you need to help the water best extract the active ingredients from the plant.

When you buy your plants at the herbal shop, they usually have already undergone this crushing step, so that even the inexperienced can go home and make their own herbal tea.

This is why I advised you in the section on preservation to buy often and in small quantities from the herbalist shop. If you have chosen a good place, with quick recycling of goods, you will still always have fairly fresh and active herbs. Buying large quantities of already crushed herbs, on the other hand, would soon leave you with an "old" and increasingly less active product in your home.

To weigh your herbs you have two alternatives, you can either buy a precision scale that allows you to measure even very small doses, or use the rough diagram you see below. The scales will be useful for weighing the weekly amount and also the daily amount, but if you buy the herbs the herbalist will already give you the bag with the weekly amount, so it may be an unnecessary purchase. In either case, you can get by just fine with the table for approximations.

For Dried Chopped Herbs

Amount	Correspondence in oz
1 large handful	About 1.8 oz
1 fistful	About 1.1 oz
1 tablespoon	About 0.4 oz
1 dessert spoon	About 0.2 oz
1 teaspoon	About 0.1 oz
1 three-finger pinch	About 0.07 oz

For Liquid Doses

Amount	Correspondence in us gal
1 mug	0,066
1 glass	0,031
1 teacup	0,026
1 coffee cup	0,013
1 shot glass	0,0079

Amount	Correspondence in us gal
1 tablespoon	0,0039
1 dessert spoon	0,0026
1 teaspoon	0,0013

Well, at this point you know almost everything there is to know about the herbs that go into your herbal teas. Before we move on, I'd like to take a look with you at the best times to harvest the various parts of the various plants. That way you will have the complete picture and we can proceed to the uses of the various plants and the useful remedies for your body and your health.

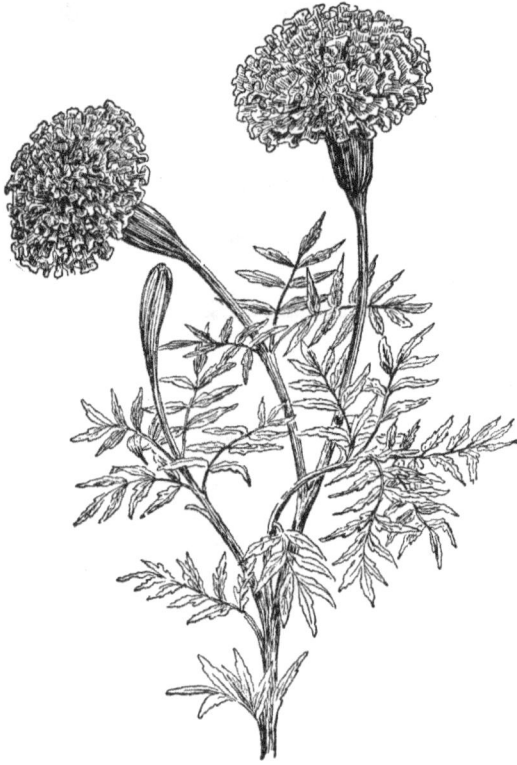

Marigold

What Part of the Plant to Harvest and When

In this chapter, you will find 5 handy grids for identifying the best time to harvest each part of a plant you may need. You will find the most popular plants in those grids to speed up your harvesting process. For those that are missing, you can use the information learned in the previous chapter to determine the best time to harvest.

In the following, you will see that some plants are indicated several times and in different sections. This is because several parts of many plants can be exploited at different times of the year and, depending on the picking time, they will present different strengths on the various active ingredients they contain.

You will find 5 grids divided into the four harvest seasons plus one for those plants and plant parts that can be harvested year-round. Each grid contains the name of the plants in the first column, the part of the plant to be harvested in that season, and the best months to do that harvesting.

Plant Parts That Can Be Harvested All Year Round

Plant	Part of the Plant
Spruce	Bark
Aloe Vera	Leaves
Cherry Tree	Bark
Eucalyptus	Leaves
Lemon	Fruits
Medlar	Leaves
Olive Tree	Leaves
Elm	Bark
Plantain	Roots
Maritime Pine	Needles
Lodgepole Pine	Resin
Parsley	Leaves
Rosemary	Leaves & Flowers
Sage	Leaves

Plant Parts That Can Be Harvested in Spring

Plant	Part of the Plant	Best Time
Spruce	Resin, needles, and gems	March & April
Sorrel	Leaves	March & April
Garlic	Leaves	April & May
Holly	Whole plant	April
Marshmallow	Leaves	June

Plant	Part of the Plant	Best Time
Dill	Leaves	From April to July
Angelica	Leaves	May & June
Mugwort	Leaves	May & June
Asparagus	Buds and woody stems	April & May
Absinthe	Leaves	From March to June
Burdock	Leaves	April & May
Basil	Whole plant	From April to September
Birch	Bark and sap	March & April
Hawthorne	Buds	March & April
Borage	Leaves	April & May
Marigold	Flowers	From April to July
Caper	Buds and Roots	From the 15th of May to the 3rd of June
Artichoke	Leaves	March
Chestnut	Leaves	April & May
Chestnut	Bark	May
Cherry	Flowers and leaves	April & May
Watercress	Leaves and stems	From May to September
Tarragon	Leaves	From March to September
Chives	Bulbs and leaves	April & May
Wild Fennel	Leaves	From April to October
Strawberry	Leaves	June
Ash	Bark	April

Plant	Part of the Plant	Best Time
Juniper	Leaves	From April to October
Raspberry	Flowers	May & June
Hops	Buds	April & May
Mint	Leaves	June
Red Cranberry	Whole plant	From May to August
Black Cranberry	Leaves	From April to June
Olive Tree	Bark	February and March
Meadowsweet	Leaves	May & June
Nettle	Whole plant	May & June
Poppy	Petals and capsules	May & June
Maritime Pine	Sap	From February to October
Lodgepole Pine	Bark, needles, and gems	February and March
Parsley	Flowers	From May to October
Primrose	Flowers and leaves	April & May
Blackthorne	Leaves and flowers in bud	April & May
Gooseberry	Buds	April & May
Robinia	Flowers	April & May
Oak	Leaves	June
Oak	Bark from tender branches	April & May
Arugula	Leaves	From May to October
Rue	Leaves	From May to August
Willow	Tips with flower	From May to August
Willow	Leaves	March & April

Plant	Part of the Plant	Best Time
Sage	Tips with flower	From May to August
Elderberry	Flowers	From April to June
Soapworts	Leaves and stems	From March to May
Dandelion	Buds and leaves	March & April
Linden	Bark	April & May
Thyme	Tips with flowers and leaves	From May to July
Valerian	Roots and wooden stems	March & April
Veronica	Whole plant	From May to July
Violet	Flowers and leaves	March & April

Plant Parts That Can Be Harvested in Summer

Plant	Part of the Plant	Best Time
Spruce	Leaves	From June to August
Yarrow	Whole plant	July and August
Garlic	Bulb	September
Alchechengi	Fruits and leaves	August and September
Laurel	Leaves	July and August
Marshmallow	Flowers	July
Dill	Seeds	September
Angelica	Seeds and stems	June and July
Arnica	Roots	September
Arnica	Flowers and leaves	From June to August
Mugwort	Flowers	July and August

Plant	Part of the Plant	Best Time
Wormwood	Tips with flowers	From July to September
Basil	Whole plant	From April to September
Birch	Leaves	From June to September
Hawthorn	Fruits	September
Borage	Flowers	June
Marigold	Flowers	From April to July
Chamomile	Tips with flowers	July and August
Artichoke	Roots	July and August
Artichoke	Tips with flower	End of June
Chicory	Leaves	From June to September
Cherry	Fruits	June and July
Watercress	Leaves and stems	From May to September
Tarragon	Flowers	July and August
Tarragon	Leaves	From March to September
Chives	Flowers	July and August
Eyebright	Whole plant	From July to September
Fig	Fruits	From June to September
Wild Fennel	Seeds	July and August
Wild Fennel	Leaves	From April to September

Plant	Part of the Plant	Best Time
Wild Fennel	Roots	From September to November
Cornflower	Whole plant	July and August
Strawberry	Fruits	July and August
Ash	Leaves and seeds	End of June
Mulberry	Fruits	July and August
Mulberry	Branches	June
Juniper	Leaves	From April to September
Raspberry	Fruits	August and September
Lavender	Flowers	June and July
Hops	Female flowers and cones	August and September
Majoram	Tips with flowers	August and September
Majoram	Leaves	July and August
Mallow	Flowers and leaves	From June to September
Almond	Seeds	July and August
Melissa	Tips with flowers and leaves	From June to September
Pomegranate	Flowers	July and August
Mint	Tips with flowers	July and August
Mint	Leaves	June
Red Cranberry	Whole plant	From May to September
Red Cranberry	Fruits	August and September
Black Cranberry	Fruits	August and September
Myrtle	Leaves	August

Plant	Part of the Plant	Best Time
Walnut	Leaves	July and August
Meadowsweet	Flowers	From July to September
Oregano	Flowers and leaves	July and August
Nettle	Whole plant	May and June
Plantain	Seeds	From June to August
Maritime Pine	Sap	From February to October
Parsley	Flowers and leaves	From May to September
Red Currant	Fruits	July and August
Rose Hip	Flowers in bud, leaves, and fruits.	August and September
Arugula	Leaves	From May to September
Rue	Leaves	From May to August
Willow	Bark	From June to September
Sage	Tips with flowers	From May to August
Elderberry	Leaves	July and August
Linden	Flowers	June and July
Thyme	Branches with flowers and leaves	From May to August
Jerusalem Artichoke	Tuber	August and September
Clover	Tips with flowers	From July to September
Gooseberry	Fruits	July and August
Verbena	Tips with flowers	From July to September

Plant	Part of the Plant	Best Time
Veronica	Whole plant	From May to August

Plant Parts That Can Be Harvested in Fall

Plant	Part of the Plant	Best Time
Sorrel	Roots	October
Laurel	Berries	October and November
Marshmallow	Roots	October
Angelica	Roots	September and October
Burdock	Roots	October
Chestnut	Fruits	October and November
Chestnut	Bark	October
Chicory	Roots	September and October
Arbutus	Whole plant	From October to January
Wild Fennel	Roots	September and October
Wild Fennel	Leaves	From April to October
Strawberry	Roots	September and October
Mulberry	Leaves	October
Gentian	Roots	From September to November
Juniper	Berries	October and November
Juniper	Leaves	From April to October
Horse Chestnut	Seeds and Bark	October and November

Plant	Part of the Plant	Best Time
Licorice	Roots	September and October
Apple	Fruits	From September to November
Pomegranate	Seeds and Bark from the roots	From September to November
Myrtle	Fruits	From October to January
Medlar	Fruits	November and December
Walnut	Fruits	October
Hazel	Fruits and leaves	September and October
Olive Tree	Bark	October and November
Meadowsweet	Roots	September and October
Maritime Pine	Buds and pine nuts	September and October
Parsley	Roots	October and November
Parsley	Flowers	From May to October
Primrose	Roots	October and November
Blackthorne	Fruits and bark from the newest branches	October and November
Gooseberry	Roots	October and November
Rhubarb	Wooden Stems	October and November
Horseradish	Roots	October and November
Oak	Acorns	September and October
Soapwort	Roots	October and November

Plant	Part of the Plant	Best Time
Rowan	Fruits and leaves	From July to October
Dandelion	Roots	September and October
Jerusalem Artichoke	Flowers	October and November
Valerian	Wooden stems and roots	October and November

Plant Parts That Can Be Harvested in Winter

Plant	Part of the Plant	Best Time
Hawthorn	Bark	February
Mulberry	Roots	January and February
Olive	Fruits	From November to January
Elderberry	Bark	January and February

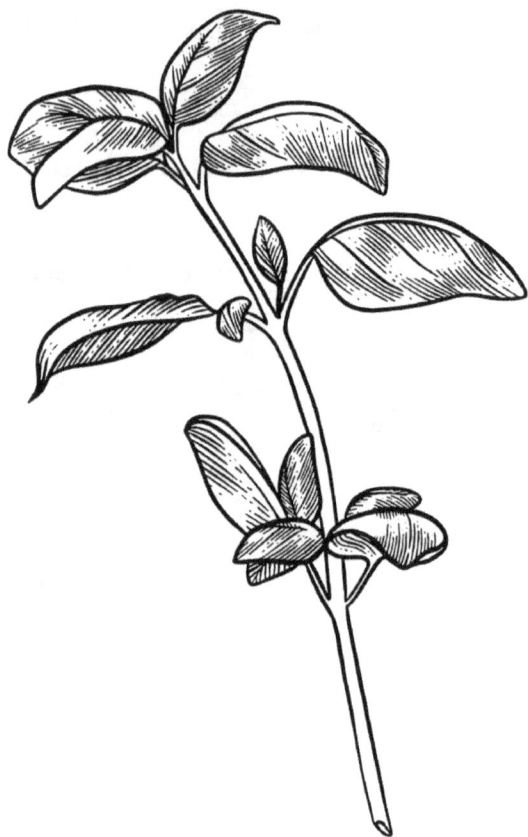

Basil

Your Stash

It should now be clear enough how to start putting together your herbal stockpile to keep on hand. You should have decided whether to buy the herbs from the herbalist shop or whether you should devote yourself to the various steps of harvesting, storing, or, even, growing them.

In the following chapter, I would like to list the main herbs you may need to have on hand. For each, I will list the major characteristics and best uses, so that you can choose which ones to include in your supply. Obviously, each plant has multiple benefits, I will only list the main ones to simplify. You will find most of the herbs in the list below in the herbal remedies in the next two chapters, and there, based on their use and combinations with other plants, you will understand the whole sphere of benefits.

Before I leave you with the list, I would like to remind you that each part of the same plant should be stored separately because some remedies may prefer a single part, while others the whole plant. For example, one remedy may require only the mallow flowers, while another also requires the leaves, and having the various parts separate allows you to combine them at the appropriate time or use them individually when needed.

Here are the plants to consider for your personal supply:

- **Aloe:** Digestion and proper absorption of food.

- **Angelica:** Anti-pain and digestive.

- **Artichoke:** Helps eliminate toxins and deflate the abdomen.

- **Ash:** Excellent against joint pain.

- **Basil:** Draining, depurative and diuretic.

- **Birch:** Anti-inflammatory, anti-bacterial, draining, and useful against cellulite.

- **Blueberry:** It is an excellent astringent, antihemorrhagic, and very useful in cases of diarrhea.

- **Borage:** Useful against fever and pain, with strong detoxifying, depurative, and diuretic properties.

- **Burdock:** Antiseptic, healing, detoxifying, depurative, and diuretic.

- **Chamomile:** Antiseptic, sedative, antibacterial, and anti-inflammatory.

- **Cherry:** Counteracts water retention and thins fat deposits. Most useful as an anti-inflammatory and diuretic.

- **Chestnut:** Lymph-draining, expectorant, and emollient for the respiratory tract.

- **Chicory:** Helps relieve an irritable colon, it is useful in cases of frequent constipation and flatulence.

- **Cinnamon:** Antiseptic, antibacterial, stimulant, and digestive.

- **Cloves:** Stimulate circulation, help against headaches and exhaustion because of their tonic properties, and aid digestion.

- **Coriander:** Antiseptic. Useful for flu, dizziness, digestion, and in cases of fatigue.

- **Cornflower:** Decongestant and anti-inflammatory, good for tired or irritated eyes.

- **Currant:** Diuretic, depurative, antiallergic, anti-inflammatory, and antioxidant. It is very useful for blood circulation given its antiplatelet property.

- **Dandelion:** Promotes digestion, stimulates diuresis, and helps the liver get rid of excess toxins.

- **Elderberry:** It helps blood circulation, keeps skin beautiful and young, promotes bowel regularity, and is diuretic and detoxifying.

- **Elm:** Disinflames mucous membranes, heals, and is an excellent astringent.

- **Eyebright:** Antiseptic, decongestant, and anti-allergic, especially concerning the eye area.

- **Eucalyptus:** Primarily balsamic and expectorant, with anti-inflammatory and antiseptic properties.

- **Gentian:** Digestive, anti fermentative, and stimulates gastric function.

- **Green Anise:** Relaxes intestinal muscles and prevents intestinal fermentation.

- **Hawthorn:** Promotes dilation of arteries and tones heart muscles.

- **Heather:** Anti-inflammatory especially for the urinary tract, antiseptic, and astringent.

- **Holly:** Helps against fever and flu.

- **Horsetail:** Mineralizing for bones, teeth, hair, and nails.

- **Hops:** Helps with anxiety, restlessness, agitation, and insomnia. It has a sedative action.

- **Laurel:** Helps digestion, swelling of the abdomen, and expulsion of gas in the intestines.

- **Lavender:** Antiseptic, antidepressant, sedative, and tonic for the nervous system.

- **Lemon balm:** Sedative and excellent for muscle spasms. The combination of these two characteristics makes it excellent for relaxing and combating anxiety and stress.

- **Licorice:** Protects the gastric mucosa, and is anti-inflammatory, digestive, and depurative.

- **Linden:** Relaxes the nervous system and muscles in general. It is also an excellent diuretic and detoxifier.

- **Mallow:** Anti-inflammatory, especially for the mouth area, diuretic, and mildly laxative.

- **Marigold:** Heals inflammation and is an excellent antioxidant.

- **Marjoram:** Promotes hormone balance, regularizes the cycle, and is a useful antioxidant.

- **Meadowsweet:** Very useful for flu, fever, and headache. Sedative, diuretic, and anti-inflammatory.

- **Mint:** Thirst-quenching, refreshing, depurative, and digestive.

- **Myrtle:** Strengthens the immune system, is a useful astringent for diarrhea, and is an excellent anti-inflammatory, especially for gums and hemorrhoids.

- **Nettle:** Diuretic and anti-inflammatory, especially useful for joint and muscle pain.

- **Oak:** Astringent, antiviral, anti-inflammatory, and disinfectant. It is a very useful treatment for diarrhea.

- **Olive:** It is useful for regulating and controlling blood pressure, cholesterol, and blood sugar.

- **Orange:** Possesses sedative properties, useful for anxiety, stress, and poor quality sleep.

- **Oregano:** It promotes gastric juices by aiding digestion. It is also soothing and analgesic.

- **Plantain:** Excellent for treating inflammation, especially of the mouth, throat, and airways. It is also emollient and sedative, so it is very useful for coughs and sore throats.

- **Pine:** Balsamic and antiseptic, it is good for colds, fevers, and inflamed airways as in coughs.

- **Rosemary:** Balsamic and anti-inflammatory. Good for coughs, colds, and inflamed throats.

- **Raspberry:** Helps the intestines perform their functions smoothly and relieves stomach pain.

- **Rue:** Excellent antimicrobial and sedative, calms the nervous system, soothes cramps, and eases pain.

- **Sage:** Stimulates appetite, aids digestion, helps respiratory inflammation, protects against microbes, and aids memory and menopausal discomfort.

- **Soapwort:** Diuretic, depurative, tonic, and expectorant.

- **Sorrel:** Depurative, laxative, and refreshing.

- **Spruce:** Helps the respiratory tract.

- **Thyme:** Relaxes the muscles, particularly those of the airways and trachea, making it very useful in cases of a loud cough. It is also antiseptic, antibacterial, and helps expel mucus.

- **Valerian:** Sedative of the nervous system, it relaxes muscles and muscle spasms, and is very useful in alleviating states of anxiety.

- **Verbena:** Protects the liver, aids digestion, and helps the nervous system fight stress.

- **Veronica:** It purifies the blood and is a diuretic, which makes it very useful for rheumatism and gout. It is also a good expectorant useful for winter discomforts such as coughs, colds, and phlegm.

- **Walnut:** Excellent astringent and very useful against fungi.

- **Wild Fennel:** Helps gastrointestinal disorders and bowel irregularity.

- **Willow:** Anti-inflammatory, analgesic, and helps eliminate fever.

- **Wormwood:** Helps the intestines, stomach, digestion, and regulates appetite.

- **Yarrow:** Helps digestion and pain from periods or colitis.

Basic Infusions to Get You Started

Now that we have seen how to prepare our herbs and organize a stash, let's start by looking at some useful infusion recipes to begin getting comfortable with this new art you are acquiring.

I recommend you start with infusions to acquire confidence in preparing and the habit of drinking. Once you feel confident enough, just dive into the remedies section and try to prepare all the other remedies. It is an easy process, but this preparation exercise will be helpful, in fact, in case of need you will be prepared in getting your remedy ready.

To prepare each infusion, you'll need to combine an equal amount of all the herbs and plants listed in the ingredients section inside a mason jar and keep it stored where light does not filter (or in an airtight non-transparent container).

To prepare 1 cup of infusion, you will need to heat the water and steep 1 dessert spoon of herbal mixture in it. Remember that the water should, by no means, reach boiling point. Let it steep for 7 to 10 minutes, using a timer so as not to let it steep too much or too little. After the appropriate time has passed, strain through a strainer, add a little honey (if you want to sweeten it), and drink your infusion. Always remember not to drink your infusion too hot.

Infusion to Improve Digestion

When to consume it: Consume the infusion after meals to aid digestion. It can also be effective to consume it half an hour before meals.

Ingredients:

- Leaves: Mint, Lemon Balm, Thyme, and Sage.

- Flowers: Chamomile, Cornflower, and Yarrow.

Properties: It contains mainly bitter plants that stimulate digestion and help manage the feeling of heaviness that often happens after meals.

Infusion to Improve Sleep

When to consume: One cup at night before going to bed.

Ingredients:

- Leaves: Lemon Balm, and Mallow.

- Flowers: Mallow, Lavender, Hops, and Chamomile.

Properties: Promotes natural relaxation and helps the body to fall asleep, thanks to the mix of plants with relaxing properties.

Winter Infusion

When to consume: Three cups throughout the day

Ingredients:

- Leaves: Thyme, Horehound, Plantain, and Mallow.

- Flowers: Marigold, Mallow, Yarrow, and Elderberry.

Properties: It mainly contains plants with strong anti-congestant power and, therefore, it is very useful in winter, when colds, flu, and cough often occur.

Draining Infusion

When to consume it: Three cups throughout the day.

Ingredients:

- Leaves: Mallow, Nettle, and Horsetail.

- Flowers: Mallow, Elderberry, and Yarrow.

Properties: It helps the body eliminate excess fluids.

Energy Infusion

When to consume: You should consume one cup in the morning at breakfast. It can also be consumed as a substitute for tea for morning tea drinkers.

Ingredients:

- Leaves: Sage, Nettle, Mint, and Horsetail.

- Flowers: Cornflower and Marigold.

Properties: It provides tone and energy. It is, therefore, especially useful during seasonal changes, when one is feeling a little sluggish, and for those who need energy for physical activity either outdoors or in the gym.

Healing Herbal Remedies

In this chapter, you will find simple and useful remedies to prepare at home, to provide relief and treat mild and common ailments and minor injuries. It will become a helpful handbook of natural medicine for you.

You will find a remedy for all those problems too mild to be brought to the doctor's attention. All those minor ailments that cannot be considered real diseases and for which medicines would be too strong and heavy a remedy.

With herbs you can heal skin problems, digestive problems, problems with fatigue and low energy, minor wounds and excoriations, poor quality of sleep, a mild cold, elimination of excess fluids, and many other minor discomforts.

These natural remedies can also be an excellent support to traditional medicine therapies. One should never rule out the use of actual medicines, but natural remedies are often a good supplement to alleviate symptoms and enjoy a bit of well-being by soothing the symptoms.

The remedies are organized alphabetically according to the discomfort they go to alleviate or prevent. For easy reference, simply scroll through the table of contents or pages following the alphabetical order of each section to locate the right herbal remedy to solve your problem.

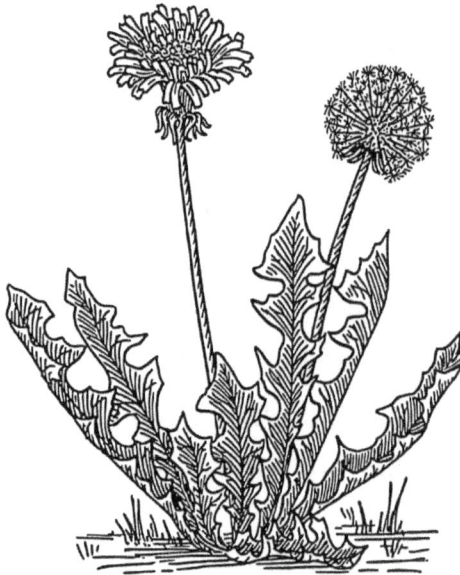

Dandelion

Remedies to Relief or Prevent Minor Conditions

Acne and Pimples

Yarrow Infusion

Ingredients:

- 2 cups of water

- 0,7 oz of dried Yarrow flowers

Preparation:

1. Heat the water thoroughly without bringing it to a boil.

2. Pour the water over the dried flowers in a teapot.

3. Let steep for 10 minutes, then strain to drink.

Consumption: Drink 3 cups a day, one in the morning on an empty stomach, one after lunch, and one after dinner.

Calendula Infusion

Ingredients:

- 2 cups of water

- 0,7 oz of dried Marigold flowers

Preparation:

1. Heat the water thoroughly without bringing it to a boil.

2. Pour the water over the dried flowers in a teapot.

3. Let steep for 10 minutes, then strain to drink.

Consumption: Drink 2 cups a day, at your preferred time of day.

Mixed Infusion

Ingredients:

- 2 cups of water

- 0,35 oz of dried Sage

- 0,35 oz dried Thyme

- 0,35 oz of dried Lavender

Preparation:

1. Heat the water thoroughly without bringing it to a boil.

2. Pour the water over the dried herbs in a teapot.

3. Let steep for 7 minutes, then strain to drink.

Consumption: Split the infusion into 3 portions and consume it after each meal (breakfast, lunch, and dinner).

Soapwort Decoction

Ingredients:

- 4 cups of water

- 2,8 oz of dried Soapwort roots

Preparation:

1. Bring the water to a boil and add the roots.

2. Boil for 12 minutes, let cool, and then strain through a strainer.

3. Pour the decoction into a stoppered bottle, where you will keep it for use.

Use: Soak a cotton ball with the decoction and use the cotton to cleanse your face, in the morning when you get up and at night before bed.

Burdock Decoction

Ingredients:

- 4 cups of water

- 2,4 oz of dried Burdock roots

Preparation:

1. Bring the water to a boil, then add the dried roots.

2. Boil for 20 minutes, let cool, and then strain through a strainer.

3. Transfer the decoction to a stoppered bottle, where you will keep it for use.

Use: Using a cotton swab, spread the decoction directly on each pimple. Repeat 2 times a day.

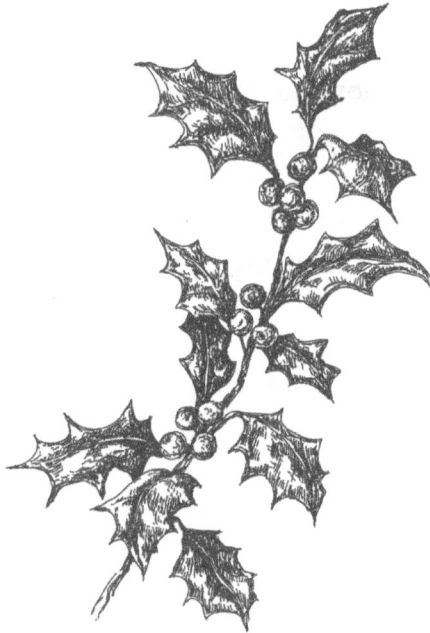

Holly

Anemia

Certain foods, when implemented into one's daily routine, can help the symptoms and discomforts of this circumstance. These are apricots, cherries, chard, spinach, asparagus, carrots, and parsley.

Thyme Infusion

Ingredients:

- 4 cups of water

- 1 oz of dried Thyme (leaves + flowers)

Preparation:

1. Heat the water very well, without bringing it to a boil.

2. Put the dried Thyme in the bottom of a teapot and pour in the hot water.

3. Let it steep for 10 minutes, then strain, and pour into a pitcher with a lid.

Consumption: Split the infusion into 3 portions and consume it away from meals.

Walnut Infusion

Ingredients:

- 4 cups of water

- 0,7 oz of dried Walnut leaves

Preparation:

1. Heat the water very well, without bringing it to a boil.

2. Put the dried leaves in the bottom of a teapot and pour in the hot water.

3. Let it steep for 15 minutes, then strain, and place in a jug with a lid.

Consumption: Split the infusion into 3 portions and consume it before each meal.

Nettle Decoction

Ingredients:

- 2 cups of water

- 0,7 oz dried Nettle, finely chopped (leaves + stems)

Preparation:

1. Bring the water to a boil, then add the Nettle.

2. Boil the decoction for 5 minutes, then turn off the heat and let it steep for 15 minutes.

3. Strain, then pour the strained decoction into a jug with a lid.

Consumption: Drink 2 cups a day, whenever you like.

Horsetail Decoction

Ingredients:

- 2 cups of water

- 0,7 oz of dried Horsetail

Preparation:

1. Bring the water to a boil, then add the Horsetail.

2. Boil the decoction for 10 minutes, then strain.

3. Pour the strained decoction into a pitcher with a lid.

Consumption: Drink 2 cups a day, whenever you like, for about 3 consecutive weeks.

Anxiety & Stress

Mixed Infusion

Ingredients:

- 3 cups of water

- 0,7 oz of dried Hawthorn

- 0,35 oz of dried Linden

- 0,35 oz of dried Mint

- 0,35 oz of dried Yarrow

Preparation:

1. Mix the herbs inside a Mason jar.

2. Warm the water, without bringing it to a boil.

3. Put 3 teaspoons of the dried herbs mixture in the bottom of a teapot and then pour the hot water over them.

4. Let it steep for 10 minutes and then strain to drink.

5. Keep it in a thermal container so that it stays warm throughout the day.

Consumption: Drink your infusion 3 times a day, away from meals, preferably a little warm. The infusion should be consumed in rotation for two weeks on then one week off, then again two weeks on and one week off, and so on.

Mixed Infusion

Ingredients:

- 4 cups of water

- 0,7 oz of dried Peppermint

- 0,7 oz of dried Chamomile

- 0,7 oz of dried Linden

- 0,7 oz of dried Verbena

Preparation:

1. In a mason jar, mix all the herbs.

2. Heat the water very well, without bringing it to a boil.

3. Put 4 teaspoons of the dried herbs mixture in the bottom of a teapot and then pour the hot water over them.

4. Let it steep for 7 minutes and then strain through a strainer so that it is ready to drink.

Consumption: Drink it throughout the day, whenever you feel a sense of anxiety coming on.

Marjoram Infusion

Ingredients:

- 1 cup of water

- 0,3 oz of chopped Marjoram leaves

Preparation:

1. Heat the water very well, without bringing it to a boil.

2. Put the dried herbs in the bottom of a teapot and then pour the hot water over it.

3. Let it steep for 5 minutes and then strain through a strainer so that it is ready to drink.

Consumption: Drink 2 cups during the day, preparing it just before you want to consume it.

Mixed Macerate

Ingredients:

- 4 cups of 40° alcohol

- 3,5 oz of dried Lemon Balm

- 0,9 oz of dried Orange peel

- 0,3 oz of Nutmeg

- 0,3 oz of Cloves

- 0,3 oz of Cinnamon

- 0,15 oz dried Angelica root

- 0,15 oz of dried Coriander

Preparation:

1. Place all the herbs and alcohol in a container suitable for steeping, cover it with the lid provided, and be sure to place it in a dimly lit place away from direct sunlight.

2. Let the macerate steep for 15 days.

3. Strain it and transfer it to a glass bottle with an airtight stopper. Store the bottle away from light.

Consumption: To consume, pour 1 tablespoon of macerate into a cup of water. You can sweeten it with a little honey if the alcohol makes the flavor too intense for you. Drink a cup when you feel anxious or stressed.

Valerian Macerate

Ingredients:

- 2 cups of water

- 1,7 oz of fresh Valerian roots (0,8 oz of dried roots, if fresh ones are unavailable)

Preparation:

1. Place the water and herbs in a steeping container, cover it with the lid provided, and steep in a dimly lit place away from direct light.

2. Let it macerate for 12 hours.

3. Strain it well and then pour it into a glass bottle with an airtight stopper. Keep the bottle away from light.

Consumption: Drink 2 coffee cups a day, whenever you like, throughout the day.

Relaxing Bath

Ingredients:

- 1 bathtub of very hot water

- 1 oz of dried Chamomile

- 1 oz of dried Orange blossom

- 1 oz of dried Linden

- 1 oz of dried Mallow

- 1 oz of dried Lemon Balm

- 1 oz of dried Lavender

- 1 oz of dried Hops

Preparation:

1. Fill the bathtub with very hot water.

2. Put all the herbs in a light cotton handkerchief or inside a gauze, then close it tightly with a knot. You need to make an infusion bag so that the herbs do not come out. Dip the bag into the tub and let it steep for 30 minutes.

3. Squeeze the bag well so that it releases all the juices of the herbs into the water. Get into the bath and soak for 20 minutes.

4. Get up slowly, rinse with lukewarm water, and then get out. A relaxing bath is ideal before going to bed.

TIP: To prevent the bath from becoming cold, you can fill the bath with hot water only half full and add the other half with hot water after the infusion time, just before getting in. The ideal way to relax is to bathe in fairly warm water, so choose the best option to ensure a good temperature.

Arthritis

Certain foods are especially helpful in providing relief from this discomfort. The most indicated ones are leeks, artichokes, cabbage, cucumbers, garlic, lemon, grapefruit, apple, cherries, strawberries, currants, and grapes.

Ash Infusion

Ingredients:

- 3 cups of water

- 1 oz of dried Ash leaves

Preparation:

1. Heat the water very well, without bringing it to a boil.

2. Put the dried leaves in the bottom of a teapot and then pour the hot water over them.

3. Let it steep for 10 minutes, strain through a strainer, and let it cool before consuming the first cup. Store the rest in a jug with a lid to consume during the day.

Consumption: Drink 3 cups a day, whenever you like.

Cherry Decoction

Ingredients:

- 2 cups of water

- 0,9 oz of dried Cherries

Preparation:

1. Bring the water to a boil and add the cherries.

2. Boil for 10 minutes on low heat, then strain.

3. Drink a cup and keep the second one covered with a lid to drink it during your day.

Consumption: Drink 2 cups a day, for 3 consecutive weeks.

Linden Wraps

Ingredients:

- 4 cups of water

- 1.8 oz of dried Linden flowers

Preparation:

1. Boil the water, then turn off the heat.

2. Add the linden blossoms and leave to infuse until the water has cooled completely.

3. Strain and store in a glass bottle with a stopper.

Usage: Use the remedy to make compresses on areas affected by discomfort. Soak gauze or thin cotton cloth to apply the remedy directly to the needed zone.

Meadowsweet Bath

Ingredients:

- 4 cups of water

- 1.1 oz of dried Meadowsweet (flowers + leaves)

Preparation:

1. Heat the water very well, without bringing it to a boil.

2. Put the meadowsweet in the bottom of the teapot and then pour the hot water over it.

3. Let it steep for 10 minutes and then strain through a strainer. Pour into a glass bottle with a stopper.

Usage: Pour the infusion into the hot water in a bathtub just before getting in and soaking yourself. You can also use the remedy you obtained to take local baths only in the affected areas. For example, you could soak your feet and ankles or hands and wrists, in a small basin.

Asthma

In the case of asthma, there are several foods whose consumption is very helpful, for example, pollen, parsley, barley, lettuce, cabbage, carrot, garlic, and onion.

Lavender Infusion

Ingredients:

- 3 cups of water

- 1 oz of dried Lavender flowers

Preparation:

1. Heat the water very well, without bringing it to a boil.

2. Put the lavender in the bottom of a teapot and then pour the hot water over it.

3. Let it steep for 5 minutes and then strain through a strainer. Pour into a pitcher with a lid.

Consumption: Drink the 3 cups during the day, at your preferred times.

Valerian Infusion

Ingredients:

- 3 cups of water

- 1.2 oz of dried Valerian roots

Preparation:

1. Heat the water very well, without bringing it to a boil.

2. Put the Valerian in the bottom of a teapot and then pour the hot water over it.

3. Let it steep for 10 minutes and then strain through a strainer. Pour into a pitcher with a lid.

Consumption: Drink the 3 cups during the day, at your preferred times.

Infusion Hyssop

Ingredients:

- 1 cup of water

- 0,5 oz of dried Hyssop

Preparation:

1. Heat the water very well, without bringing it to a boil.

2. Put the Hyssop in the bottom of the teapot and then pour the hot water over it.

3. Let it steep for 10 minutes, then strain through a strainer and drink.

Consumption: Drink one cup a day, at your preferred time of day.

Oregano Decoction

Ingredients:

- 4 cups of water

- 1 oz of dried Oregano (leaves + flowers)

Preparation:

1. Bring the water to a boil and add the Oregano.

2. Boil for 10 minutes, then strain and add a little honey to make it more palatable.

3. Keep in a jug with a lid.

Consumption: Drink 3 cups during the day, at your preferred times.

TIP: Remember that when you prepare decoctions a fairly big part of the water gets lost through evaporation and filtering. Follow each remedy's ingredients and instructions and drink the amount poured in your jug, split in the number of portions recommended in the consumption instructions.

Bad breath

Bad breath can be caused by various conditions, usually related to the digestive system. As an immediate solution, you could chew fresh or dried leaves of wild mint or peppermint. As a longer-term solution try the following remedies.

Mixed Infusion

Ingredients:

- 2 cups of water

- 0,3 oz of dried Lemon Balm

- 0,15 oz of dried Rosemary

- 0,15 oz of Gentian

- 0,15 oz of Chamomile

Preparation:

1. Heat the water very well, without bringing it to a boil.

2. Put the dried herbs in the bottom of a teapot and pour in the hot water.

3. Let it steep for 4 minutes, then strain to drink.

Consumption: Drink 2 cups throughout the day, preferably after breakfast and after lunch, for at least 20 consecutive days.

TIP: As you should consume the remedy for at least 20 days, you can mix a bigger amount of the herbs in a mason jar. Make sure you follow the proportions between herbs when you mix them. This way you will only have to pick up a full teaspoon of mixture for each cup you are preparing.

Thyme Infusion

Ingredients:

- 4 cups of water

- 1,7 oz of dried Thyme flowering tops

Preparation:

1. Heat the water, without it reaching a boil.

2. Put the Thyme in the bottom of a teapot and pour the hot water over them.

3. Let it steep for 10 minutes and then strain.

4. This infusion is not to be drunk but used for rinses, so pour it into a practical use container.

Usage: Use the infusion for mouth rinses. It should be used frequently throughout the day, as a kind of mouthwash.

Myrtle Decoction

Ingredients:

- 4 cups of water

- 1 oz of dried Myrtle leaves

Preparation:

1. Bring the water to a boil and then add the dried Myrtle leaves.

2. Boil the decoction for 10 minutes, let it cool and then strain through a strainer.

3. Pour the strained decoction into a stoppered bottle, where you will keep it for use.

Use: Use the decoction to rinse your mouth at least three or four times a day. Hold it in your mouth for about 30 seconds, rinsing as if it were mouthwash.

Back pain

Linden Bark Decoction

Ingredients:

- 4 cups of water

- 1 oz of dried Linden bark

Preparation:

1. Bring the water to a boil then add the bark.

2. Simmer for 15 minutes on low heat and then strain.

3. Pour it into a jug with a lid, where you will keep it for 2 days in a fresh place.

Consumption: Get 4 portions out of your decoction. Drink 2 cups a day for 2 days.

Verbena Wraps

Ingredients:

- Water, just enough

- 1 egg white

- 0,7 oz of dried Verbena leaves

Preparation:

1. Blanch the Verbena leaves in a little hot water for a couple of minutes.

2. With a slotted spoon, retrieve the verbena leaves and add them to the egg white. Stir vigorously.

3. Put the mixture in a clean cotton cloth or washcloth.

Use: Make sure the compress is not burning hot and apply it to the area affected by the pain, keeping the mixture inside the washcloth.

Bad skin

Skin Glow Decoction

Ingredients:

- 4 cups of water

- 1.4 oz of dried Sorrel roots

Preparation:

1. Bring the water to a boil then add the roots.

2. Boil for 5 minutes, then turn off the heat and let it steep for another 5 minutes.

3. Strain and pour the decoction into a jug with a stopper.

Consumption: Drink the decoction divided into 3 cups, to be consumed at any time during the day. You should consume the decoction for 3 consecutive weeks.

Skin Tonic Decoction

Ingredients:

- 4 cups of water

- 1,7 oz of dried Beard roots

Preparation:

1. Bring the water to a boil then add the roots.

2. Boil for 20 minutes and then strain.

3. Pour it into a jug with a stopper, where you will keep it
    for the day.

Consumption: Drink the decoction divided into 3 cups, to be
consumed whenever you like throughout the day. You must
consume the decoction for 3 consecutive weeks.

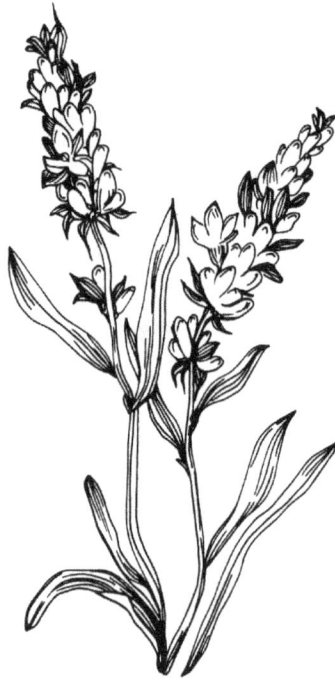

Lavender

Bronchitis

Eucalyptus Infusion

Ingredients:

- 1 cup of water

- 0,2 oz dried Eucalyptus

Preparation:

1. Heat the water very well, without bringing it to a boil.

2. Put the Eucalyptus in the bottom of a teapot, then pour the hot water over it.

3. Let it steep for 7 minutes, then strain through a strainer and drink.

Consumption: Drink one cup a day, whenever you feel like it.

Plantain Infusion

Ingredients:

- 1 cup of water

- 0,2 oz of dried Plantain

Preparation:

1. Heat the water very well, without bringing it to a boil.

2. Put the Plantain in the bottom of a teapot, then pour the hot water over it.

3. Let it steep for 10 minutes, then strain through a strainer and drink.

Consumption: Drink one cup a day, whenever you feel like it.

Elderberry Infusion

Ingredients:

- 1 cup of water

- 0,2 oz of dried Elderberry

Preparation:

1. Heat the water very well, without bringing it to a boil.

2. Put the Elderberry in the bottom of a teapot, then pour the hot water over it.

3. Let it steep for 10 minutes, then strain through a strainer and drink.

Consumption: Drink one cup a day, whenever you feel like it.

Mixed Decoction

Ingredients:

- 2 cups of water

- 1 fresh Apple, with peel, diced

- 0,2 oz dried Licorice

Preparation:

1. Bring the water to a boil and add the Licorice and the apple diced.

2. Boil for 20 minutes, then strain and drink, when lukewarm.

Consumption: Drink one cup a day, preferably before going to bed.

Burns

For mild burns:

Meadowsweet Decoction

Ingredients:

- 4 cups of water

- 1,7 oz of dried Meadowsweet

Preparation:

1. Bring the water to a boil then add the Meadowsweet.

2. Boil for 10 minutes on low heat and then strain.

3. Pour into a bowl and let it cool down.

Usage: Use the decoction to create tablets by soaking gauze or cotton. Apply the decoction-soaked compresses to the burn.

For deeper burns, it is better to create fresh compresses by finely chopping on the spot flowers, fruits, or herbs. Here are the best alternatives.

Potatoes: Slice some potatoes, after carefully cleaning them of soil. Place the freshly cut slices directly on the burn. Turn the slices after a few minutes and replace them when they have begun to lose their moist appearance and have warmed up.

Pumpkin: Finely chop or blend some fresh pumpkin pulp, after removing the rind and seeds. Apply the resulting mixture directly to the burn and leave it on for a few minutes. Repeat several times throughout the day, always freshly chopping the pumpkin at the time of application.

Ivy: Finely chop some fresh ivy leaves, after washing them thoroughly. Apply the resulting mixture directly to the burn and leave it on for a few minutes. Repeat the operation several times throughout the day, always freshly chopping the leaves at the time of application.

Carrots: Finely chop the pulp of a raw carrot, after washing it thoroughly. Apply the resulting mixture directly to the burn and leave it on for a few minutes. Repeat several times throughout the day, always freshly chopping the carrots at the time of application.

Marigold: Finely chop some fresh marigold flowers, after making sure they are well cleaned. Apply the resulting mixture directly to the burn and leave it on for a few minutes. Repeat several times throughout the day, always freshly chopping the flowers at the time of application.

Burps and farts

For Burps:

Mixed Infusion

Ingredients:

- 1 cup of water

- 0,5 oz of dried Chamomile

- 0,3 oz of dried Coriander

- 0,3 oz of dried Mint

- 0,5 oz of dried Green Anise

Preparation:

1. In an airtight glass jar, mix the herbs together.

2. Heat the water very well, without bringing it to a boil.

3. Put 1 teaspoon of the herb mixture in the bottom of a cup and pour the hot water over it.

4. Let it steep for 10 minutes, then strain through a strainer.

Consumption: Drink the infusion 3 times a day, 15-20 minutes before meals, preparing it just before consumption.

Fennel Infusion

Ingredients:

- 1 cup of water

- 0,5 oz of dried Green Anise

- 0,5 oz of dried Fennel

Preparation:

1. In an airtight glass jar, mix the Anise and the Fennel.

2. Heat the water very well, without bringing it to a boil.

3. Put half a teaspoon of the herb mixture in the bottom of the cup and pour the hot water over it.

4. Let it steep for 10 minutes, then strain through a strainer.

Consumption: Drink the infusion 3 times a day, just after meals, preparing it just before consumption.

For farts:

Mixed Infusion

Ingredients:

- 1 cup of water

- 1 oz of dried Chamomile

- 1 oz of dried Fennel

- 0,7 oz of dried Mint

- 0,7 oz of dried Juniper berries

Preparation:

1. In an airtight glass jar, mix together the herbs.

2. Heat the water well, without bringing it to a boil.

3. Put 1 teaspoon of the herb mixture in the bottom of the cup and pour the hot water over it.

4. Let it steep for 15 minutes, then strain and drink.

Consumption: The infusion should be drunk after meals. It should be consumed bitter, drunk hot but not boiling, and should be prepared shortly before consumption.

Caries Prevention

Useful in preventing cavities is Alliaria. You will need to chew a fresh leaf of it on a fairly regular basis.

Catarrh

Sage Infusion

Ingredients:

- 3 cups of water

- 0,7 oz of dried Sage leaves

Preparation:

1. Heat the water well without bringing it to a boil.

2. Put the sage leaves in the bottom of a teapot, after crushing them a little, then pour the hot water over them.

3. Let it steep for 15 minutes, then strain through a strainer and pour into a pitcher with a lid.

Consumption: Drink 3 cups a day, whenever you like throughout the day.

Cellulite

Providing relief for cellulite are all those plants that help fluid elimination and those with a tonic effect. This applies to both herbal teas and nutrition. You can therefore also benefit from your diet by eating grapes, apples, oranges, seaweed, artichokes, onions, parsley, and dandelion.

Infusion to Eliminate Extra-Fluids

Ingredients:

- 2 cups of water

- 0,35 oz of dried Elderflowers

Preparation:

1. Heat the water well, without bringing it to a boil.

2. Put the flowers in the bottom of a teapot and pour the hot water over them.

3. Let it steep for 7 minutes then strain immediately through a strainer.

Consumption: Drink 2 cups of infusion, one in the morning and one in the evening.

Detox and Deflating Infusion

Ingredients:

- 3 cups of water

- 0,7 oz of dried Artichoke leaves

Preparation:

1. Heat the water well, without bringing it to a boil.

2. Put the leaves in the bottom of a teapot and pour the hot water over them.

3. Let it steep for 10 minutes then strain through a strainer and transfer to a pitcher with a lid.

Consumption: Drink 3 cups of infusion throughout the day. One cup in the morning on an empty stomach, one cup in the afternoon, and one in the evening after dinner, just before bedtime.

Detox Decoction

Ingredients:

- 2 1/2 cups of water

- 0,2 oz of dried Nettle leaves

- 0,2 oz of dried Birch leaves

- 0,2 oz of dried Yarrow

- 0,2 oz of dried Chicory

- 0,35 oz of dried Burdock root

Preparation:

1. Bring water to a boil and add the herbs.

2. Boil for 6 minutes, then strain and divide into 2 cups.

Consumption: Drink one cup in the morning and one in the evening.

Reactivating Decoction

Ingredients:

- 1 cup of water

- 0,35 oz of dried Birch

- 0,35 oz of dried Ash

- 0,35 oz of dried Meadow Queen

- 0,35 oz of dried Red Vine

- 0,35 oz dried Green Anise seed

Preparation:

1. In an airtight glass jar, mix together the herbs.

2. Bring the water to a boil and add 1 teaspoon of the herbs mixture.

3. Boil for 5 minutes, turn off the heat, and let steep for 10 minutes, then strain.

Consumption: Drink one cup every night just before bedtime.

Sae Oak Poultice

Ingredients:

- 4 cups of water

- 3,5 oz of whole dried tufts of Sea Oak

Preparation:

1. Bring the water to a boil, then add the sea oak.

2. Boil for 15 minutes, then turn off the heat.

3. When the decoction is well heated, but not boiling, strain it through a strainer, using your hands to drain all the juices from the removed sea oak.

4. Place the hot decoction in a fairly large bowl.

Use: Take a cotton cloth, small towel, or gauze pads and soak them in the hot liquid. Squeeze them lightly, then gently place the warm cloths on the parts affected by cellulite. Repeat the operation until the liquid is used up.

TIP: Repeat the operation at least 1 or 2 times a week. If the areas to be treated are small, you can prepare half the liquid by halving the decoction ingredients.

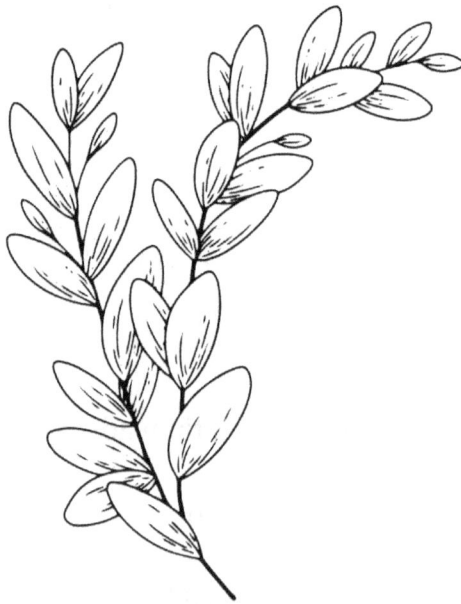

Eucalyptus

Chilblains

Decoction of White Spruce or Elderflower

Ingredients:

- 4 cups of water

- 1,7 oz of dried White Spruce

   or

- 1,2 oz of dried Elderflowers

Preparation:

1. Bring the water to a boil then add the White Spruce or Elderflower, whichever is easiest for you to get.

2. Boil for 10 minutes on low heat, turn the flame off, and put the lid on.

3. Let steep for 10 minutes before straining.

4. Pour into a bowl and let cool further if necessary. It should be hot enough, but not scalding hot.

Use: Soak your hands or feet in the decoction for at least 15 minutes.

TIP: You can use the decoctions to make washes on directly affected areas, rubbing the infusion vigorously.

Circulation

Sorrel Decoction

Ingredients:

- 4 cups of water

- 1 oz of dried Sorrel

Preparation:

1. Bring the water to a boil then add the Sorrel.

2. Boil for 10 minutes on low heat and then strain.

3. Prepare the water for the foot bath and add the decoction, making sure it is hot but not boiling, otherwise, you may scald yourself. The ideal temperature is that of the foot bath itself, which you can measure with an immersion thermometer if you want to be more accurate.

Use: Perform a foot bath of at least 15 minutes whenever you feel the need.

TIP: This foot bath is especially useful for swollen ankles or heavy legs. Usually, these discomforts are caused by poor circulation and are common in those who are on their feet for many hours, perhaps for work, such as sales clerks.

Cholesterol

Birch Infusion

Ingredients:

- 3 cups of water

- 0,7 oz of dried Birch leaves

Preparation:

1. Heat the water well, without bringing it to a boil.

2. Put the leaves in the bottom of the teapot and pour the hot water over them.

3. Let steep for 10 minutes then strain through a strainer and transfer to a pitcher with a lid.

Consumption: Drink 3 cups a day, at your preferred times of the day.

Dandelion Decoction

Ingredients:

- 3 1/2 cups of water

- 1 oz of dried Dandelion root

Preparation:

1. Bring the water to a boil, then add the Dandelion.

2. Boil for 10 minutes, then strain well and place in a jug with a lid.

Consumption: Drink 3 cups of decoction daily. The first should be consumed in the morning on an empty stomach, the other two when you prefer, throughout the day.

Mixed Decoction

Ingredients:

- 3 1/2 cups of water

- 0,5 oz of dried Ash leaves

- 0,5 oz of dried Birch bark

Preparation:

1. Bring the water to a boil, then add the ash and the birch.

2. Boil for 5 minutes, then turn off the heat and let steep for 5 minutes.

3. Strain through a strainer and pour into a jug with a lid.

Consumption: Drink 3 cups of decoction during the day, with the first one in the morning on an empty stomach and the other two when you prefer, throughout the day.

Conjunctivitis

Eyebright Decoction

Ingredients:

- 4 cups of water

- 0,5 oz of dried Eyebright

Preparation:

1. Bring the water to a boil and then add the dried Eyebright.

2. Boil the decoction for 10 minutes, let it cool, and then strain through a sieve.

3. Pour the strained decoction into a stoppered bottle, where you will keep it for use.

Use: With a cotton ball, gently cleanse the area around the affected eye. With a clean cotton ball, create a compress, soak it with the decoction, and place it for a few minutes on the eyelid of the affected eye.

Chamomile Infusion

Ingredients:

- 2 cups of water

- 0,8 oz of dried Chamomile

Preparation:

1. Heat the water well without bringing it to a boil.

2. Put the Chamomile in the bottom of the teapot and pour the hot water over it.

3. Let it steep for 20 minutes, then strain it carefully using a strainer. Place it in a bowl.

Use: With a cotton ball gently cleanse the area around the affected eye. Using a clean cotton ball, create a compress, soak it with the decoction, and place it on the eyelid of the affected eye for a few minutes.

TIP: You can also make the chamomile wash with chamomile tea in filters that they sell at the supermarket. Use 2 cups of water and two filters (or 1 cup and one filter, if the affected eye is only one) and let it steep for 10 minutes. Take out the two filters, squeeze them slightly, let them cool and place them on closed eyelids for 10-15 minutes.

Colds

Mixed Infusion

Ingredients:

- 1 cup of water

- 0,35 oz of dried Eucalyptus leaves

- 0,35 oz of dried Mallow

Preparation:

1. Heat the water very well, without bringing it to a boil.

2. Put the herbs in the bottom of a cup and pour the hot water over them.

3. Let it steep for 7 minutes, then strain through a strainer.

Consumption: Drink one cup a day, after lunch or after dinner, until symptoms have passed.

Elderflowers Infusion

Ingredients:

- 3 cups of water

- 1 oz of dried Elderflowers

Preparation:

1. Heat the water very well, without bringing it to a boil.

2. Put the herb in the bottom of a teapot and pour the hot water over them.

3. Let it steep for 10 minutes, then strain through a strainer.

4. Pour the infusion into a small pitcher with a lid.

Consumption: Drink 3 cups a day, throughout the day, whenever you prefer.

Eyebright Infusion

Ingredients:

- 1 cup of water

- 0,15 oz of dried Eyebright

Preparation:

1. Heat the water very well, without bringing it to a boil.

2. Put the Eyebright in the bottom of a cup and pour the hot water over it.

3. Let it steep for 10 minutes, then strain through a strainer.

4. Sweeten the infusion with honey.

Consumption: Drink one cup a day when you feel the symptoms.

Primerose Infusion

Ingredients:

- 2 cups of water

- 0,35 oz of dried Primrose

Preparation:

1. Heat the water very well, without bringing it to a boil.

2. Put the Primrose flowers and leaves in the bottom of a teapot and pour the hot water over them.

3. Let it steep for 10 minutes, then strain through a strainer.

4. Divide the infusion into two cups and let cool.

Consumption: Consume the two cups throughout the day between meals.

Cough

Expectorant Infusion

Ingredients:

- 1 cup of water

- 0,25 oz of dried Mallow

- Honey, to taste

Preparation:

1. Heat a cup of water well, without bringing it to a boil.

2. Put the Mallow in the bottom of the cup and pour the hot water over it. Let it steep for 10 minutes.

3. Strain and add honey to make it very sweet.

4. Keep in a cup covered with a lid.

Consumption: Drink 4 coffee cups during the day.

Expectorant Decoction

Ingredients:

- 3 1/2 cups of water

- 1 oz of dried Lungwort leaves

Preparation:

1. Bring the water to a boil, then add the dried leaves.

2. Let it boil for 10 minutes, then turn off the heat and strain.

3. Store the decoction in a jug with a lid.

Consumption: Drink 3 cups during the day.

Decoction for a Persistent or Phlegmy Cough

Ingredients:

- 2 cups of water

- 0,7 oz of dried needles of Scots Pine

Preparation:

1. Bring the water to a boil, then add the Pine needles.

2. Let it boil for 15 minutes, then turn off the heat and strain.

3. Store the decoction in a corked bottle.

Consumption: Drink several coffee cups during the day, as needed.

Mixed Infusion

Ingredients:

- 4 cups of water

- 0,5 oz of dried Thyme

- 0,5 oz of dried Mallow

- 0,5 oz of dried Mint

- 0,2 oz of dried Basil

Preparation:

1. Heat the water well, without bringing it to a boil.

2. Put the herbs in the bottom of a teapot and pour the hot water over it, let it steep for 5 minutes.

3. Strain and pour it into a pitcher with a lid.

Consumption: Drink 3 cups a day. One cup after each meal (breakfast, lunch, and dinner).

Basil Infusion for Persistent Cough

Ingredients:

- 3 cups of water

- 0,7 oz of dried Basil (leaves + flowering tops)

Preparation:

1. Heat the water well, without bringing it to a boil.

2. Put the Basil in the bottom of the teapot and pour the hot water over it, let it steep for 10 minutes.

3. Strain and pour into a pitcher with a lid.

Consumption: Drink 3 cups a day, away from meals.

Mint Infusion for Persistent Cough

Ingredients:

*   3 cups of water

*   0,7 oz of dried Mint (leaves + flowering tops)

Preparation:

1. Heat a cup of water well, without bringing it to a boil.

2. Put the Mint in the bottom of a teapot and pour the hot water over it, let it steep for 5 minutes.

3. Strain and pour into a pitcher with a lid.

Consumption: Drink 3 cups a day, away from meals.

Cystitis

To alleviate discomforts due to cystitis you can use infusions and decoctions with diuretic and depurative action, as well as the ones described underneath. Nutrition is also of extreme help in providing relief in this circumstance that causes severe discomfort. Recommended foods include pumpkin, fava beans, garlic, onion, cabbage, fennel, apples, grapes, and leeks.

Scots Pine Infusion

Ingredients:

- 1 cup of water

- 0,2 oz dried buds of Scots Pine

Preparation:

1. Heat the water well, without bringing it to a boil.

2. Put the buds at the bottom of the cup and pour the hot water over them.

3. Let steep for 20 minutes then strain through a strainer.

Consumption: Drink 1 cup a day, at your preferred time of day.

Mixed Decoction

Ingredients:

- 3 1/2 cups of water

- 0,7 oz of dried Heather flowers

- 1 oz of dried Mallow (flowers and leaves)

Preparation:

1. Bring the water to a boil, then add the herbs.

2. Boil for 10 minutes over low heat, then strain well and place in a jug with a lid.

Consumption: Drink 3 cups daily in the breaks between meals.

Cranberry Decoction

Ingredients:

- 3 1/2 cups of water

- 1,4 oz of dried Cranberry

Preparation:

1. Bring the water to a boil, then add the Cranberry.

2. Boil for 5 minutes over low heat, then strain well and place in a jug with a lid.

Consumption: Drink 3 cups daily away from meals.

Dandruff

Chestnut Infusion

Ingredients:

- 4 cups of water

- 2.1 oz of dried Chestnut leaves

Preparation:

1. Heat the water well, without bringing it to a boil.

2. Put the leaves in the bottom of the teapot and pour the hot water over them.

3. Let it steep for 10 minutes, then strain and put it in a bottle with the cap where you will keep it for use.

Use: Make sure the infusion is well chilled before using. Apply it to the head's skin 3 times a week, rubbing in like a lotion without rinsing it.

TIP: Using the same method of preparation and the same amounts, you can substitute dry parsley leaves for chestnut leaves. The resulting infusion should be poured over the skin as an additional rinse after shampooing. If you wash your hair daily alternate its use with the chestnut infusion. If you don't wash your hair daily use it before applying the chestnut infusion.

Diabetes

Some herbs and plants help alleviate the discomfort that diabetes causes by providing some relief. In addition to decoctions and infusions, it is helpful to add the following to one's diet (check with your doctor first if this food suits you): garlic, cabbage, oats, artichokes, raw onions, corn, green beans, lentils, walnuts, hazelnuts, blueberries, dandelion, and soybeans.

Sage Infusion

Ingredients:

- 3 cups of water

- 0,7 oz of dried Sage leaves

Preparation:

1. Heat the water well without bringing it to a boil.

2. Put the Sage in the bottom of a teapot and pour the hot water over it.

3. Let it steep for 10 minutes, then strain and pour into a jug with a lid.

Consumption: Drink 3 cups daily at your preferred times.

Nettle Infusion

Ingredients:

- 2 cups of water

- 0,7 oz of dried Nettle

Preparation:

1. Heat the water well without bringing it to a boil.

2. Put the Nettle in the bottom of a teapot and pour the hot water over it.

3. Let it steep for 15 minutes, then strain and pour into a jug with a lid.

Consumption: Drink 2 cups daily, at your preferred times.

Agrimony Infusion

Ingredients:

- 3 cups of water

- 1 oz of dried Agrimony flowers and leaves

Preparation:

1. Heat the water well without bringing it to a boil.

2. Put the Agrimony in the bottom of a teapot and pour the hot water over it.

3. Let it steep for 10 minutes, then strain and pour into a jug with a lid.

Consumption: Drink 3 cups daily, at your preferred times.

Blueberry Decoction

Ingredients:

- 2 1/2 cups of water

- 0,5 oz of dried Blueberry leaves

- 0,2 oz of dried Blueberry

Preparation:

1. Bring the water to a boil, then add the dried Blueberry.

2. Boil the decoction for 5 minutes, then strain and pour into a jug with a lid.

Consumption: Drink 2 cups throughout the day, away from meals.

Diuresis, Purification, and Water Retention

Purifying Infusion

Ingredients:

- 3 cups of water

- 1 oz of dried Meadowsweet (flowers and leaves)

Preparation:

1. Heat the water well without bringing it to a boil.

2. Put the Meadowsweet in the bottom of a teapot and pour the hot water over it.

3. Let it steep for 10 minutes, then strain and pour into a jug with a lid.

Consumption: Drink t 3 cups daily, at your preferred times.

Diuretic Decoction

Ingredients:

- 4 1/2 cups of water

- 1,2 oz of dried Crabgrass roots

Preparation:

1. Bring the water to a boil, then add the dried Crabgrass.

2. Boil the decoction for 10 minutes, then strain and pour into a jug with a lid.

Consumption: Drink 4 cups daily, at your preferred times.

Birch Infusion

Ingredients:

- 3 cups of water

- 1 oz of dried Birch leaves

Preparation:

1. Heat the water well without bringing it to a boil.

2. Put the leaves in the bottom of a teapot and pour the hot water over them.

3. Let it steep for 15 minutes, then strain and pour into a jug with a lid.

Consumption: Drink 3 cups daily on breaks between meals.

Dandelion Decoction

Ingredients:

- 3 1/2 cups of water

- 1,4 oz of dried Dandelion roots

Preparation:

1. Bring the water to a boil and then add the Dandelion root.

2. Simmer the decoction for 10 minutes on low heat.

3. Let it steep in the stew for 2 hours, then strain and pour into a jug with a lid.

Consumption: Drink 3 cups daily, 15 minutes before eating breakfast, lunch, and dinner.

Infusion to Eliminate Water Retention

Ingredients:

- 3 cups of water

- 1,5 oz of dried Red Currant leaves

Preparation:

1. Heat the water well without bringing it to a boil.

2. Put the leaves in the bottom of a teapot and pour the hot water over them.

3. Let it steep for 5 minutes, then strain and pour into a jug with a lid.

Consumption: Drink 3 cups throughout the day, at times of your choice.

Diarrhea and Intestinal Disorders

In case of diarrhea, it is helpful to consume tea with lemon juice. Diarrhea leads to high fluid loss, and tea with lemon juice helps to balance this loss.

Infusion for Colitis

Ingredients:

- 1 cup of water

- 0,7 oz gr of dried Lavender

- 0,7 oz of dried Marjoram

- 0,7 oz of dried Mallow

Preparation:

1. In an airtight glass jar, mix together the herbs.

2. Heat the water well without bringing it to a boil.

3. Put 1 teaspoon of the herb mixture in the bottom of the cup and pour the hot water over it.

4. Let it steep for 10 minutes, then strain and drink.

Consumption: Drink 2 cups a day after meals, preparing it just before consumption. It should be consumed for 3 weeks a month.

Infusion for Diarrhea

Ingredients:

- 1 cup of water

- 0,2 oz of dried Green Anise

Preparation:

1. Heat the water well without bringing it to a boil.

2. Put the Anise in the bottom of the cup and pour the hot water over it.

3. Let it steep for 10 minutes, then strain and drink.

Consumption: Drink 2 cups a day, preparing it just before consumption.

Decoction for Diarrhea

Ingredients:

- 2 1/2 cups of water

- 1 oz of dried Elm bark

Preparation:

1. Bring the water to a boil, then add the bark.

2. Simmer the decoction for 20 minutes on low heat.

3. Strain, pour into a jug with a lid, and let it cool.

Consumption: Consume 2 cups throughout the day.

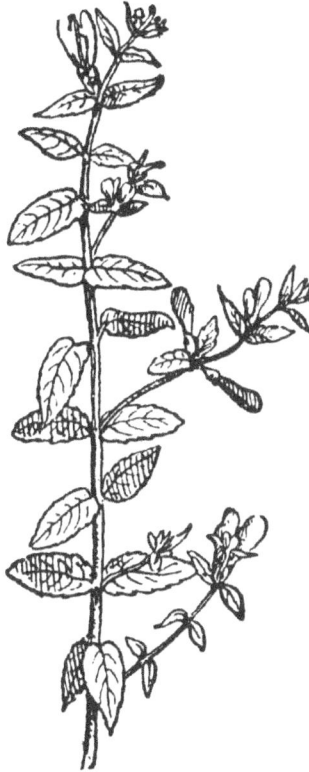

Mint

Digestion

There are numerous foods that, consumed during a meal, help digestion, for example, parsley, celery, fennel, mint, artichokes, oranges, and grapes.

Infusion to Aid Digestion

Ingredients:

- 1 cup of water

- 0,5 oz of dried Mint

- 0,5 oz of dried Fennel seeds

- 0,3 oz of dried Chamomile

- 0,3 oz of dried Lemon Balm

Preparation:

1. In a glass jar with an airtight seal, mix the herbs together.

2. Heat the water well without bringing it to a boil.

3. Put 1 tablespoon of the blended herbs in the bottom of the cup and pour the hot water over it.

4. Let it steep for 10 minutes, then strain and drink.

Consumption: The infusion should be consumed after a meal and should be drunk bitter.

Digestive and Depurative Infusion

Ingredients:

- 1 cup of water

- 0,15 oz of dried Verbena

Preparation:

1. Heat the water well without bringing it to a boil.

2. Put the verbena in the bottom of the cup and pour the hot water over it.

3. Let it steep for 10 minutes, then strain and drink.

Consumption: The infusion should be consumed after a meal and should be drunk bitter.

Laurel Infusion

Ingredients:

- 1 cup of water

- 2/3 dried Laurel leaves

Preparation:

1. Heat the water well without bringing it to a boil.

2. Put the Laurel leaf in the bottom of the cup and pour the hot water over it.

3. Let it steep for 10 minutes, then strain and drink.

Consumption: The infusion should be consumed after a meal and should be drunk bitter.

Anti-Stomach-Acidity Infusion

Ingredients:

- 1 cup of water

- 0,7 oz of dried Chamomile

- 0,7 oz of dried Linden

- 0,7 oz of dried Bitter Orange blossoms

Preparation:

1. In an airtight glass jar, mix all the herbs.

2. Heat the water well without bringing it to a boil.

3. Put 1 teaspoon of the herb mixture in the bottom of the cup and pour the hot water over it.

4. Let it steep for 10 minutes, then strain and drink.

Consumption: The infusion should be consumed after a meal and should be drunk bitter. For best results over time, consume it for 2 weeks and repeat the following month, if necessary.

Anti-Stomach-Acidity Decoction

Ingredients:

- 4 cups of water

- 0,7 oz of dried Licorice root

- 0,7 oz of dried Mallow

- 0,7 oz of dried Lemon Balm

- 0,7 oz of dried Chamomile

Preparation:

1. Bring the water to a boil, then add the Mallow and the Licorice.

2. Let boil for 10 minutes, over low heat.

3. Turn off the heat, add the Lemon Balm and Chamomile and let cool for 10 to 12 minutes with the herbs infused.

4. Strain and pour into a jug with a stopper.

Consumption: Drink several cups during the day, depending on the intensity of the discomfort.

Infusion for Digestion (if you have eaten too much)

Ingredients:

- 1 cup of water

- 0,15 oz of dried Verbena

- 0,15 oz of dried Green Anise

- 0,15 oz of dried Linden

Preparation:

1. Heat the water well, without bringing it to a boil.

2. Put the herbs in the bottom of the cup and pour the hot water over them.

3. Let it steep for 7 minutes, then strain.

Consumption: Drink it after a meal to aid digestion.

Infusion for Cramps Due to Poor Digestion

Ingredients:

- 1 cup of water

- 0,7 oz of dried Mint

- 0,7 oz of dried Lemon Balm

Preparation:

1. Heat the water well, without bringing it to a boil.

2. Put the herbs in the bottom of the cup and pour the hot water over them.

3. Let it steep for 10 minutes, then strain.

Consumption: Drink it at the onset of discomfort to ease digestion.

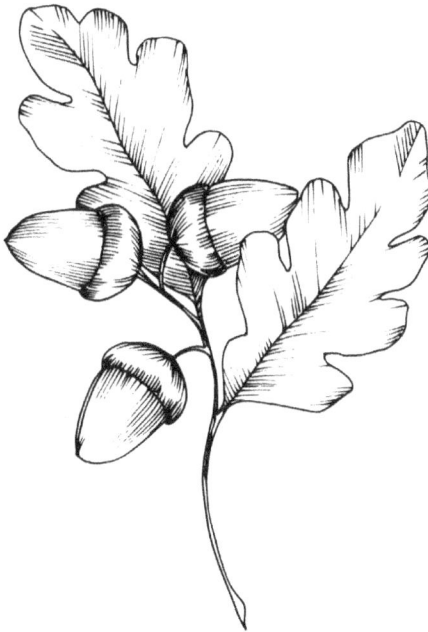

Oak

Female Intimate Itching

Mixed Decoction

Ingredients:

- 4 cups of water

- 2,1 oz of dried Oak bark

- 1 oz of dried Lavender

- 1 tablespoon of organic apple cider vinegar

Preparation:

1. Bring the water to a boil then add the oak bark.

2. Boil for 5 minutes on low heat and then turn off the heat.

3. Add the lavender and the apple cider vinegar and cover with a lid. Let steep for about half an hour, until the decoction has cooled.

4. Strain and pour into a bowl.

Use: Using a sprinkler, apply the decoction to the itchy intimate area. Do not rinse when finished, just gently wipe the affected area.

TIP: It is very helpful to apply a 100% natural marigold cream to the outer area after applying the decoction.

Lavender Decoction

Ingredients:

- 4 cups of water

- 1,7 oz of dried Lavender flowers

Preparation:

1. Bring water to a boil then add the Lavender.

2. Boil for 5 minutes over low heat, let cool, and then strain.

3. Pour into a glass bottle with a stopper to store the decoction.

Use: Using a special sprinkler, make an internal wash every morning. Do not rinse, just gently dry the affected area.

TIP: To make the wash even more effective, it would be ideal to warm the decoction to body temperature before irrigation. Use an immersion thermometer to measure the temperature and avoid overheating the decoction.

Fever

Eucalyptus Infusion

Ingredients:

- 3 cups of water

- 0,7 oz of dried Eucalyptus leaves

Preparation:

1. Heat the water well, without bringing it to a boil.

2. Put the leaves in the bottom of a teapot and pour the hot water over them.

3. Let it steep for 10 minutes, then strain and place in a pitcher where you will keep it for the day.

Consumption: Drink 3 cups during the day.

Wormwood Infusion

Ingredients:

- 1 cup of water

- 0,15 oz of dried Wormwood flowering tops

Preparation:

1. Heat the water well, without bringing it to a boil.

2. Put the wormwood in the bottom of the teapot and pour the hot water over it.

3. Let it steep for 10 minutes, then strain and drink.

Consumption: Drink one cup a day.

Chestnut Infusion

Ingredients:

- 3 cups of water

- 0,7 oz of dried Chestnut leaves

Preparation:

1. Heat the water well, without bringing it to a boil.

2. Put the leaves in the bottom of the teapot and pour the hot water over them.

3. Let it steep for 10 minutes, then strain and place in a pitcher where you will keep it for the day.

Consumption: Drink 3 cups a day, at your leisure.

Ash Decoction

Ingredients:

- 3 1/2 cups of water

- 1 oz of dried Ash bark

Preparation:

1. Bring the water to a boil, then add the bark.

2. Let it boil for 15 minutes, strain it, and put it in a jug with a stopper to store it throughout the day. This is a rather bitter decoction and you may need to sweeten it with a little honey. Do this while the decoction is still warm enough for the honey to dissolve.

Consumption: Drink 3 cups a day at your preferred times.

Flu

It is very useful to use the remedies from the earliest symptoms to speed up the healing process as much as possible.

Mixed Infusion

Ingredients:

- 1 cup of water

- 0,7 oz of dried Licorice

- 0,7 oz of dried Borage

- 0,7 oz of dried Linden

- 0,7 oz of dried Elderflowers

Preparation:

1. In a jar with an airtight seal, mix the dried herbs together.

2. Heat 1 cup of water very well, without bringing it to a boil.

3. Put a tablespoon of the herb mix in the bottom of the cup and pour the hot water over it.

4. Let it steep for 10 minutes, then strain through a strainer.

5. Drink the infusion hot.

Consumption: Consume 2 cups daily, away from meals. Brew it each time, just before drinking.

This decoction is very useful not only as an anti-flu, but also in cases of mild fever, cough, and phlegm.

Marigold Decoction

Ingredients:

- 1 1/2 cup of water

- 0,2 oz of dried Marigold flowers

Preparation:

1. Bring the water to a boil then add the Marigold.

2. Boil for 5 minutes and then strain immediately.

3. Drink the decoction hot, but not boiling.

Consumption: Drink two cups a day, whenever you like. Prepare it each time just before consuming.

Frigidity

Chestnut Infusion

Ingredients:

- 1 cup of water

- 0,5 oz dried flowering Sage

Preparation:

1. Heat the water well, without bringing it to a boil.

2. Put the Sage in the bottom of the cup and pour the hot water over it.

3. Let it steep for 10 minutes, then strain and drink.

Consumption: Drink 1 cup every night.

Gastritis

Chamomile

Ingredients:

- 1 cup of water

- 0,2 oz of dried Chamomile

- Freshly squeezed juice of half an organic lemon

Preparation:

1. Heat the water well, without bringing it to a boil.

2. Put the Chamomile in the bottom of the cup and pour the hot water over it.

3. Let it steep for 15 minutes.

4. Add lemon juice, then strain and drink.

Consumption: Drink 2 cups a day when the ailment occurs. Drink it lukewarm and brew it just before consumption.

Hair Loss Prevention

A strong contribution to hair loss prevention can be made by diet. The most useful foods are oats, nettle, almonds, walnuts, millet, watercress, and brewer's yeast.

Basil Concentrate Infusion

Ingredients:

- 4 cups of water

- 5,3 oz of fresh Basil leaves (2,7 oz of dried leaves, if fresh ones are unavailable)

Preparation:

1. Heat the water well, but do not bring it to a boil.

2. Put the leaves in the bottom of a teapot and pour the hot water over them.

3. Let it steep for 20 minutes, then crush the basil leaves well before straining.

4. Pour into a bottle with a stopper, where you will keep it for use.

Use: Rub the infusion into the scalp 3 times a week.

Mixed Decoction

Ingredients:

- 4 cups of water

- 0,9 oz of dried Burdock

- 0,9 oz of dried Rosemary

- 0,9 oz of dried Thyme

Preparation:

1. Bring the water to a boil and add the dried herbs.

2. Boil for 15 minutes, then turn off the heat and let steep for 10 minutes.

3. Strain the decoction and keep it in a bottle with a stopper.

Use: Use the decoction to rub the scalp 2 times a week.

Headache

Linden & Orange Infusion

Ingredients:

- 1 cup of water

- 0,1 oz of dried Linden flowers

- 0,1 oz of dried Orange leaves

Preparation:

1. Heat the water well without bringing it to a boil.

2. Put the flowers and leaves in the bottom of the cup and pour the hot water over them.

3. Let it steep for 5 minutes, then strain through a strainer before drinking.

Consumption: Drink it hot before going to bed. Be careful to drink it hot and not boiling so you don't get burned.

Jasmine Infusion

Ingredients:

- 1 cup of water

- 0,2 oz of dried Jasmine flowers

Preparation:

1. Heat the water well, without bringing it to a boil.

2. Put the flowers in the bottom of the cup and pour the hot water over them.

3. Let it steep for 10 minutes then strain through a strainer before drinking.

Consumption: Drink it hot before going to bed. Be careful to drink it hot and not boiling so you don't get burned.

Hemorrhoids

Elderberry Infusion

Ingredients:

- 4 cups of water

- 1,7 oz of dried Elderflowers

Preparation:

1. Heat the water well without bringing it to a boil.

2. Put the Elderflowers in the bottom of the teapot and pour the hot water over them.

3. Let it steep for 10 minutes, then strain and pour into a bowl.

Use: Use the infusion to wash the affected area several times throughout the day. You can also soak some cotton or gauze, creating a compress, and apply it to the affected area, leaving it on for a few minutes. You can repeat the procedure 2 or 3 times a day.

Mallow Decoction

Ingredients:

- 4 cups of water

- 1,7 oz of dried Mallow

Preparation:

1. Bring the water to a boil, then add the Mallow.

2. Boil for 2 minutes.

3. Let steep for 15 minutes then strain and place in a jug with a stopper.

Consumption: Drink 3 cups a day at your preferred times, as long as it is on an empty stomach.

TIP: It is also very useful to create mallow decoction tablets to apply directly to affected areas. All you need to do is soak some cotton or gauze and apply it to the affected area for a few minutes.

Yarrow Decoction

Ingredients:

- 4 cups of water

- 1,7 oz of dried Yarrow

Preparation:

1. Bring the water to a boil, then add the Yarrow.

2. Let boil for 10 minutes over low heat, then strain.

3. Pour the decoction into a bowl.

Use: Create compresses by soaking some cotton or gauze. Apply the compresses for a few minutes directly to the affected area. Repeat several times a day.

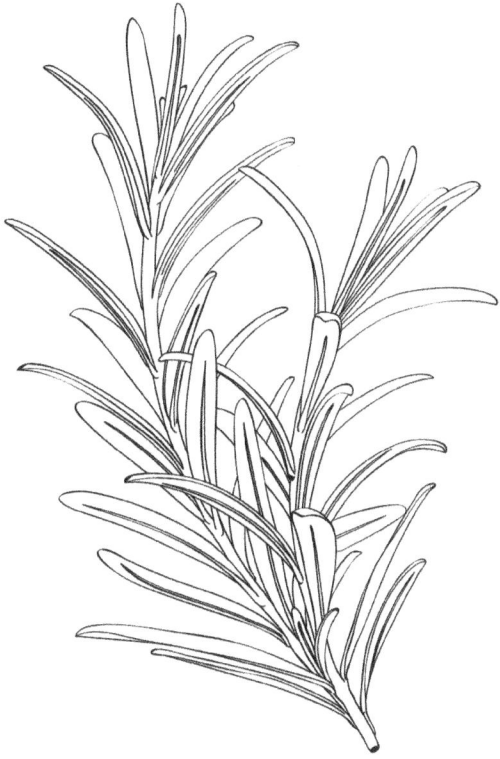

Rosemary

Herpes

Borage Infusion

Ingredients:

- 3 cups of water

- 1 oz of dried Borage flowers

Preparation:

1. Heat the water very well, without bringing it to a boil.

2. Put the flowers in the bottom of a teapot and pour the hot water over them.

3. Let it steep for 10 minutes, then strain through a strainer.

4. Pour the infusion into a pitcher with a lid.

Consumption: Consume 3 cups of infusion a day, whenever you like.

Soapwort Decoction

Ingredients:

- 2 1/2 cups of water

- 0,7 oz of dried Soapwort root

Preparation:

1. Bring the water to a boil then add the root.

2. Boil for 5 minutes then strain immediately.

Consumption: Drink 2 cups of decoction daily when you prefer.

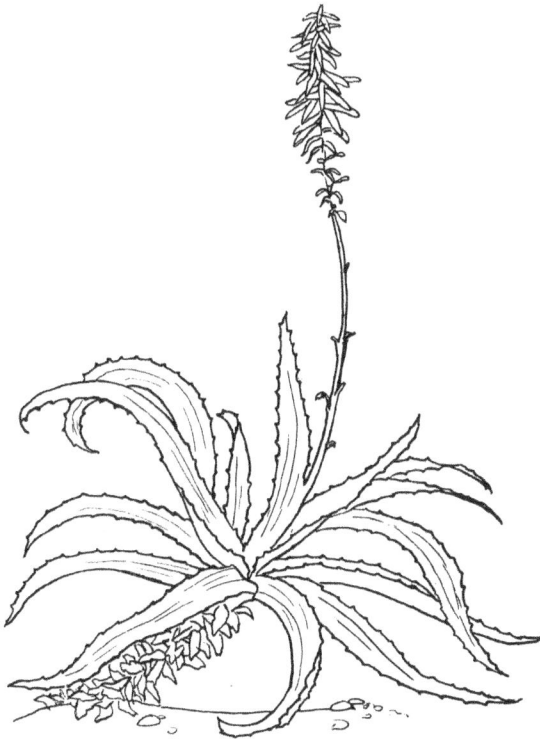

Aloe

Hiccups

The easiest natural method to quell hiccups, when they occur, is to take a teaspoon of organic freshly squeezed lemon juice. If it is too acidic for you, you can use a slightly larger spoon and add a tiny bit of honey. Absolute juice has a quicker and more effective result.

If you regularly get hiccups after meals you can drink a coffee cup of green anise infusion after each meal. You prepare it by steeping 0,7 oz of green anise seeds in 1 cup of very hot, but not boiling, water for 30 minutes. Strain the infusion before drinking it.

High Blood Pressure

The main causes of high blood pressure are poor eating habits and psychological and emotional stress. Very useful foods in helping this condition are garlic, of which one should consume one fresh clove a day, sunflower oil, rye flour, grapes, and raw spinach. As for herbs, those with calming properties and herbs that help the veins to dilate are the most useful.

For prevention:

Hawthorn Infusion

Ingredients:

- 3 cups of water

- 1 oz of dried Hawthorn flowers

Preparation:

1. Heat the water very well, without bringing it to a boil.

2. Put the flowers in the bottom of a teapot and pour the hot water over them.

3. Let it steep for 10 minutes, then strain through a strainer.

4. Pour the infusion into a pitcher with a lid.

Consumption: Drink 3 cups daily, at preferred times. The infusion should be consumed for 3 weeks each month.

Pilosella Infusion

Ingredients:

- 3 cups of water

- 1,7 oz of dried Pilosella

Preparation:

1. Heat the water very well, without bringing it to a boil.

2. Put the Pilosella in the bottom of the teapot and pour the hot water over it.

3. Let it steep for 10 minutes, then strain through a strainer.

4. Pour the infusion into a pitcher with a lid.

Consumption: Drink 3 cups daily, at your favorite times.

Periwinkle Decoction

Ingredients:

- 2 1/2 cups of water

- 0,5 oz of dried Periwinkle

Preparation:

1. Bring water to a boil then add the Periwinkle.

2. Boil for 5 minutes then strain.

3. Pour it into a jug with a stopper.

Consumption: Drink 2 cups throughout the day.

To provide relief to those already suffering from it:

Mixed Infusion

Ingredients:

- 3 cups of water

- 0,3 oz of dried Olive leaves

- 0,2 oz of dried Linden

- 0,2 oz of dried Meadowsweet

- 0,2 oz of dried Lavender

Preparation:

1. Heat the water very well, without bringing it to a boil.

2. Put the herbs in the bottom of a teapot and pour the hot water over them.

3. Let it steep for 7 minutes, then strain through a strainer.

4. Pour the infusion into a pitcher with a lid.

Consumption: Drink 3 cups during the day, after meals.

Olive Tree Infusion

Ingredients:

- 1 cup of water

- 0,15 oz of dried Olive leaves

Preparation:

1. Heat the water very well, without bringing it to a boil.

2. Place the olive tree in the bottom of the cup and pour the hot water over it.

3. Let it steep for 10 minutes, then strain through a strainer.

4. Drink it hot, but not boiling.

Consumption: Drink 1 cup in the morning on an empty stomach.

TIP: In the evening, before going to bed, you can put 5 dried olive leaves in a glass of water. Let them macerate overnight and in the morning on an empty stomach drink the cold macerate. It is a great summer alternative to infusion.

Insect Bites

Lemon or green-stemmed onion both help for insect bites, depending on the circumstances.

Bee or wasp sting: In this case, you must rub the swollen and reddened part of the bite with the green stalk of the onion. If, however, the sting has remained in the bite, it must be extracted, and in this case, once removed the bite should be rubbed with a slice of lemon.

Spider sting: In this case, one must rub the swollen and reddened part of the sting with a clove of onion.

Irritated or Inflamed Skin

Periwinkle Infusion

Ingredients:

- 1 cup of water

- 0,2 oz of dried Periwinkle leaves

Preparation:

1. Heat the water well without bringing it to a boil.

2. Put the Periwinkle leaves in the bottom of a cup and pour the hot water over it.

3. Let it steep for 10 minutes, then strain and pour into a bowl. Allow cooling well.

Use: Use the infusion to perform washes on affected areas of the skin. You can also soak some cotton or gauze with the infusion and apply it directly to the affected areas.

Itching

From atopic dermatitis (eczema):

Veronica Decoction

Ingredients:

- 4 cups of water

- 1 oz of dried Veronica

Preparation:

1. Bring the water to a boil then add the Veronica.

2. Boil for 10 minutes and then strain.

3. Pour it into a bottle with a stopper, where you will keep it for future use.

Use: Make a compress with the decoction at room temperature by soaking gauze or some cotton and applying it to affected areas that cause itching. Repeat several times throughout the day.

Blueberry Decoction

Ingredients:

- 4 cups of water

- 1,7 oz dried Blueberry (berries and leaves)

Preparation:

1. Bring the water to a boil then add the Blueberry.

2. Boil for 10 minutes and then strain.

3. Pour it into a bottle with a stopper, where you will keep it for future use.

Use: Use the decoction at room temperature to wash the itchy areas 2 times a day.

Sedge Decoction

Ingredients:

- 2 1/2 cups of water

- 10,35 oz of dried Sedge root

Preparation:

1. Bring the water to a boil then add the root.

2. Boil for 10 minutes and then strain.

3. Pour it into a jug with a stopper.

Consumption: Drink 2 cups whenever you like throughout the day.

Itching from other causes:

Plantain Infusion

Ingredients:

- 4 cups of water

- 1,7 oz of dried Plantain leaves

Preparation:

1. Heat the water very well, without bringing it to a boil.

2. Put the leaves in the bottom of a teapot and pour the hot water over them.

3. Let it steep for 10 minutes, then strain through a strainer.

4. Pour the infusion into a bowl and let it cool.

Use: Use the infusion several times a day to make frequent washes to itchy parts.

Mullein Decoction

Ingredients:

- 4 cups of water

- 2,1 oz of dried Mullein leaves

Preparation:

1. Bring the water to a boil then add the leaves.

2. Boil for 10 minutes on low heat and then strain.

3. Pour into a bowl and let it cool.

Use: Use the decoction to make frequent washes throughout the day in areas that cause itching.

Lack of Appetite & Scarce Appetite

Eating raw tomatoes before a meal can prove very helpful in developing an appetite. Gooseberry juice is also very helpful. Consume 1 glass in the morning on an empty stomach. If you like you can consume a second glass later in the day.

Hunger-Stimulating Infusion

Ingredients:

- 1 cup of water

- 0,2 oz of dried Eyebright

Preparation:

1. Heat the water well, without bringing it to a boil.

2. Put the Eyebright in the bottom of the cup and pour the hot water over it.

3. Let steep for 10 minutes, then strain and place in a cup with a lid.

Consumption: Drink 1 coffee cup before each meal.

Valerian Macerate

Ingredients:

- 4 cups of water

- 3,5 oz of fresh Valerian roots

Preparation:

1. Chop up the roots and put them in the water.

2. Leave to macerate overnight. Strain through a colander.

3. Store in a glass bottle with a stopper.

Consumption: Drink 2 glasses of cold decoction daily, one before lunch and one before dinner.

Low Blood Pressure

Herbs with a tonic and restorative function are useful for this condition.

Lemon Balm Water for Prevention

Ingredients:

- 2 cups of alcohol at 60°

- 1,7 oz of dried Lemon Balm flowers

- 0,35 oz of dried Angelica root

- 0,2 oz of Cinnamon taken from a stick

- 10 Cloves

- The fresh peel of 1 organic lemon (do not use regular lemons because the peel is processed and full of chemicals that make it harmful)

Preparation:

1. Mix all the herbs and alcohol in an airtight glass jar.

2. Macerate for 20 days away from light, shaking the mixture once a day.

3. Strain the mixture well and store in dark glass dropper bottles.

Consumption: Consume 15 drops diluted in water 3 times a day.

Invigorating Mixed Infusion

Ingredients:

- 3 cups of water

- 0,35 oz of dried Licorice root

- 0,2 oz of dried Mint

- 0,1 oz of dried Hyssop

Preparation:

1. Heat the water very well, without bringing it to a boil.

2. Put the herbs in the bottom of a teapot and pour the hot water over them.

3. Let it steep for 7 minutes, then strain through a strainer.

4. Pour the infusion into a pitcher with a lid.

Consumption: Drink 3 cups during the day, after meals.

Memory

Iron Memory Infusion

Ingredients:

- 3 cups of water

- 1 oz of dried Lemon Balm flowers

Preparation:

1. Heat the water very well, without bringing it to a boil.

2. Put the Lemon Balm flowers in the bottom of a teapot and pour the hot water over them.

3. Let it steep for 10 minutes, then strain through a strainer.

4. Pour the infusion into a pitcher with a lid.

Consumption: Drink 3 cups during the day, at preferred times. The infusion should be consumed for 10 consecutive days each month for 3 consecutive months.

Menopause

Mixed Infusion

Ingredients:

- 1 cup of water

- 1 oz of dried Linden

- 1 oz of dried Lavender

- 1 oz of dried Hawthorn

Preparation:

1. In an airtight glass jar, mix the herbs together.

2. Heat the water well, without bringing it to a boil.

3. Put 1 tablespoon of the herb mixture in the bottom of the cup and pour the hot water over it.

4. Let it steep for 15 minutes, then strain.

Consumption: Drink 2 cups a day, throughout the day, at your leisure. Drink it lukewarm, preparing it just before consumption.

Migraines

The consumption of certain foods can be very helpful in the management of migraines. Chief among these are apple, lemon, and artichoke. Useful in trying to soothe it, however, is sniffing dried pulverized basil leaves.

Marjoram Infusion

Ingredients:

- 2 cups of water

- 0,35 oz of dried Marjoram leaves

Preparation:

1. Heat the water well, without bringing it to a boil.

2. Put the dried leaves in the bottom of the teapot and pour the hot water over them.

3. Let it steep for 10 minutes, then strain.

Consumption: Drink 2 cups throughout the day.

Motion Sickness (Car, Sea, and Plane)

Lotus Infusion

Ingredients:

- 2 cups of water

- 0,35 oz of dried Lotus flowers

Preparation:

1. Heat the water very well, without bringing it to a boil.

2. Put the flowers in the bottom of the teapot and pour the hot water over them.

3. Let it steep for 10 minutes, then strain through a strainer.

4. Pour the infusion into two separate cups. Cover the one you will not be consuming anytime soon with a lid.

Consumption: 10 days before your trip, you should consume 2 cups of the infusion daily, at your preferred times of the day.

Mouth Ulcers

To treat sores and small mouth ulcers, blueberries and their juice are most useful. The juice should be held in the mouth for at least 30 seconds before swallowing. You can chew blueberries, or use juice directly.

Mouthwash Infusion

Ingredients:

- 4 cups of water

- 1,4 oz of dried flowers of Savory

Preparation:

1. Heat the water thoroughly without bringing it to a boil.

2. Put the flowers in the bottom of a teapot and pour the hot water over them.

3. Let it steep for 10 minutes, then strain through a strainer.

4. Let the infusion cool and put it in a glass bottle with a stopper to keep it between uses.

Use: Use it daily to make rinses as you would use a mouthwash. Hold it in your mouth for at least 30 seconds and repeat it at least 3 times a day until the discomfort disappears.

Basil or Nettle Decoction

Ingredients:

- 4 cups of water

- 3,5 oz of fresh Basil leaves

  or

- 1,7 oz of dried Nettle leaves

Preparation:

1. Bring the water to a boil.

2. Add the Basil or the Nettle leaves.

3. Boil for 15 minutes if you use basil and 20 minutes if you use nettle, then strain.

4. Let the decoction cool down before use.

Use: Use the decoction to rinse your mouth several times a day. Hold the liquid in your mouth for at least 30 seconds, rinsing as if it were mouthwash, before spitting it out.

Nausea and Vomit

Chewing on an ice cube is very helpful to quell wheezing.

Mixed Infusion

Ingredients:

- 1 cup of water

- 1 oz of dried Chamomile flowers

- 1,7 oz of dried Valerian root

- 0,7 oz of dried flowers of Mint

Preparation:

1. In an airtight glass jar, add all the herbs and mix them together.

2. Heat the water very well, without bringing it to a boil.

3. Put 1 teaspoon of the herb mixture in the bottom of the cup and pour the hot water over it.

4. Let it steep for 20 minutes, then strain through a strainer.

Consumption: Take 1 teaspoon of the infusion every 15-20 minutes until you feel better.

Nervousness

Plants with a sedative action are very useful in calming this condition. It is also very helpful to consume apples and apricots regularly and in abundance.

Relaxing Infusion

Ingredients:

- 1 cup of water

- 0,3 oz of dried Linden flowers

- 0,5 oz of dried Orange Blossom

- 0,5 oz of dried Violet flowers

- 0,5 oz of dried Melilot

- 0,5 oz of dried Lemon Balm

- 0,5 oz of dried Valerian root

- 0,5 oz of dried Hops

- 1 teaspoon of honey

Preparation:

1. In an airtight glass jar, mix all the ingredients except the Linden flowers and create an herbal mixture.

2. Heat the water very well, without bringing it to a boil.

3. Place the Linden flowers and a teaspoon of the herbal mixture in the bottom of the cup and pour the hot water over it.

4. Let it steep for 10 minutes, then strain through a strainer.

5. Add a teaspoon of honey.

Consumption: The infusion should be drunk as hot as possible without burning yourself while drinking it. It should be prepared before drinking. Drink 2 o 3 cups daily to relieve anxiety, nervousness, and headaches.

Chamomile

Ingredients:

- 2 cups of water

- 0,7 oz of dried Chamomile flowers

Preparation:

1. Heat the water very well, without bringing it to a boil.

2. Put the Chamomile in the bottom of the teapot and pour the hot water over it.

3. Let it steep for 10 minutes, then strain through a strainer.

4. Pour the infusion into a pitcher with a lid.

Consumption: Drink 2 cups throughout the day every day.

Holly Decoction

Ingredients:

- 4 cups of water

- 1 oz of dried Holly

Preparation:

1. Bring the water to a boil then add the Holly.

2. Simmer for 10 minutes and then strain.

3. Pour it into a jug with a stopper, where you will keep it for the day.

Consumption: The decoction should be drunk cold. Drink 3 cups throughout the day.

Relaxing Bath

Ingredients:

- Water

- 1 oz of dried Linden blossoms

- 1 oz of dried Lemon Balm flowers

- 1 oz of dried Mallow flowers

- 1 oz of dried Lavender flowers

- 1 oz of dried Hop flowers

- 1 oz of dried Chamomile flowers

- 1 oz of dried Orange Blossoms

Preparation:

1. Mix the dried flowers together and create a sort of filter using gauze tightly closed at the ends. It should come out sort of like a large teabag that does not allow the flowers to leak into the water.

2. Fill about 1/3 of the bathtub with very hot water, you can also add a little boiling water for best results.

3. Add the filter you created to the water and let it steep for half an hour.

4. Wring out the filter well, remove it from the tub, and finish filling the tub with hot water. Choose the ideal temperature for you, but keep in mind that it should be warm enough to help you relax.

Use: Stay submerged in the bath for half an hour, but no less than 15 minutes. When you are done, get up from the bath very slowly and rinse with water that is not too hot, dry off, and get into bed, even if only for a half-hour rejuvenating nap. For an even more relaxing result, cover yourself with a warm blanket.

Palpitations

Woodruff Infusion

Ingredients:

- 1 cup of water

- 0,35 oz of Woodruff

Preparation:

1. Heat the water very well, without bringing it to a boil.

2. Put the Woodruff in the bottom of the cup and pour the hot water over it.

3. Let it steep for 10 minutes, then strain through a strainer.

Consumption: Drink it hot, at the time of need.

Mixed Infusion

Ingredients:

- 3 cups of water

- 0,5 oz of dried Linden

- 0,9 oz of dried Lemon Balm

- 0,5 oz of dried Verbena

- 0,35 oz of dry White Willow

Preparation:

1. Heat the water very well, without bringing it to a boil.

2. Put the herbs in the bottom of a teapot and pour the hot water over them.

3. Let it steep for 7 minutes, then strain through a strainer.

4. Pour the infusion into a pitcher with a lid.

Consumption: Drink 3 cups a day, after meals, until the discomfort subsides.

Pre- and Post-Cycle Pain, Heavy or Irregular Flows

For Period pains:

Mixed Infusion

Ingredients:

- 3 cups of water

- 1 oz of dried Chamomile

- 1 oz of dried Calendula

- 1 oz of dried Lemon Balm

- 0,7 oz of dried Yarrow

- 0,7 oz of dried Linden

Preparation:

1. In an airtight glass jar, mix all the herbs.

2. Heat the water well without bringing it to a boil.

3. Put 2 tablespoons of the herb mixture in the bottom of a teapot and pour the hot water over it.

4. Let it steep for 10 minutes, then strain and pour it into a jug with a stopper.

Consumption: Drink 3 cups a day away from meals. Start consuming the herbal tea 7 days before the supposed start date of your period and continue drinking it for 3 days after it ends.

Yarrow Infusion

Ingredients:

- 1 cup of water

- 0,2 oz of dried Yarrow

Preparation:

1. Heat the water well without bringing it to a boil.

2. Put the Yarrow in the bottom of the cup and pour the hot water over it.

3. Let it steep for 10 minutes, then strain and drink.

Consumption: Drink one cup a day, at your preferred time of day. Start 3 days before the supposed date of your period and continue until it ends.

Raspberry Infusion

Ingredients:

- 2 cups of water

- 0,9 oz of dried Raspberry leaves

Preparation:

1. Heat the water well, without bringing it to a boil.

2. Put the dried leaves in the bottom of the teapot and pour the hot water over them.

3. Let it steep for 10 minutes, then strain.

Consumption: Drink 2 cups throughout the day, at your preferred times. Consume it at least a week before the supposed start date of your period.

To regularize sparse flows:

Mixed Infusion

Ingredients:

- 1 cup of water

- 1,7 oz of dried Rue

- 1,5 oz of dried Rosemary

- 0,5 oz of dried Aloe

Preparation:

1. In an airtight glass jar, mix all the herbs.

2. Heat the water well without bringing it to a boil.

3. Put 1/2 teaspoon of the herb mixture in the bottom of the cup and pour the hot water over it.

4. Let it steep for 10 minutes, then strain and drink.

Consumption: Drink the infusion hot, not boiling, morning and evening, preparing it just before consumption. Start consuming it about 7 days before the expected start date of your period and continue until it ends.

To regularize heavy flows:

Mixed Infusion

Ingredients:

- 1 cup of water

- 1 oz of dried Chamomile

- 1 oz of dried Mint

- 1 oz of dried Valerian

- 1 oz of dried Yarrow

Preparation:

1. In an airtight glass jar, mix all the herbs.

2. Heat the water well without bringing it to a boil.

3. Put 1 teaspoon of the herb mixture in the bottom of the cup and pour the hot water over it.

4. Let it steep for 10 minutes, then strain and drink.

Consumption: Drink 1 cup of hot infusion every morning, preparing it just before consumption. Start consuming it about 7 days before the expected start date of your period and continue until it ends.

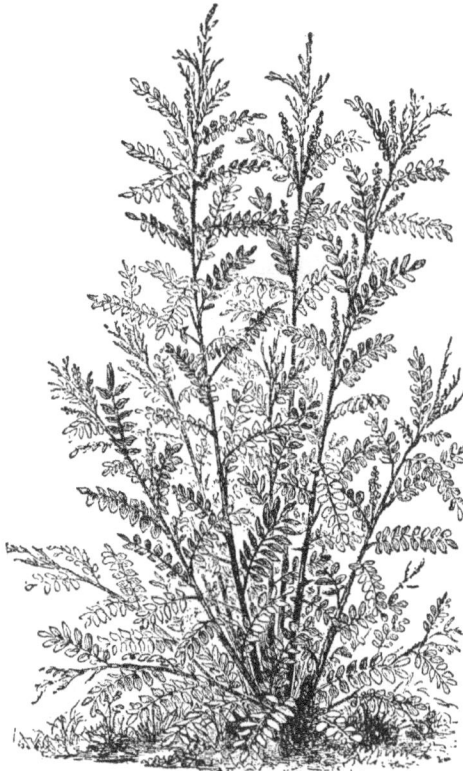

Licorice

Pharyngitis and Laryngitis

Infusion for Pharyngitis

Ingredients:

- 3 cups of water

- 0,35 oz of dried Agrimony

Preparation:

1. Heat the water well, without bringing it to a boil.

2. Put the Agrimony in the bottom of a teapot and pour the hot water over it.

3. Let it steep for 10 minutes, then strain and place in a pitcher where you will keep it for the day.

Consumption: Drink 3 cups during the day.

Infusion for Laryngitis

Ingredients:

- 3 cups of water

- 1,4 oz of dried Erysimum flowering ends

Preparation:

1. Heat the water well, without bringing it to a boil.

2. Put the Erysimum in the bottom of a teapot and pour the hot water over it.

3. Let it steep for 15 minutes, then strain and place in a pitcher where you will keep it for the day. It may turn out a little bitter, so you may want to sweeten it with a little honey before the infusion cools too much to dissolve the honey.

Consumption: Drink 3 cups throughout the day, away from meals.

Rheumatism

Linden Infusion

Ingredients:

- 2 cups of water

- 0,35 oz of dried Linden blossoms

Preparation:

1. Heat the water very well, without bringing it to a boil.

2. Put the Linden in the bottom of a teapot and pour the hot water over it.

3. Let it steep for 10 minutes, then strain through a strainer.

4. Divide the infusion into two cups and let cool.

Consumption: Consume the two cups throughout the day.

Meadowsweet Infusion

Ingredients:

- 3 cups of water

- 2 oz of Meadowsweet

Preparation:

1. Heat the water very well, without bringing it to a boil.

2. Put the Meadowsweet in the bottom of a teapot and pour the hot water over it.

3. Let it steep for 10 minutes, then strain through a strainer.

4. Pour the infusion into a jug with a stopper.

Consumption: Drink 3 cups throughout the day, every day for 3 weeks.

Black Currant Infusion

Ingredients:

- 3 cups of water

- 1,7 oz of Blackcurrant leaves

Preparation:

1. Heat the water very well, without bringing it to a boil.

2. Put the leaves in the bottom of a teapot and pour the hot water over them.

3. Let it steep for 15 minutes, then strain through a strainer.

4. Pour the infusion into a jug with a stopper.

Consumption: Drink 3 cups throughout the day, every day for 3 weeks.

Sleep and Tiredness

To improve the quality of sleep, the use of sedative relaxing plants with a mildly narcotic effect is ideal.

Mixed Infusion

Ingredients:

- 1 cup of water

- 1 oz of dried Linden

- 1 oz of dried Mallow

- 1 oz of dried Sage

- 0,5 oz of dried Verbena

- 0,5 oz of dried Bitter Orange blossom

Preparation:

1. In a mason jar, mix all the herbs together.

2. Heat a cup of water well, without bringing it to a boil.

3. Put 1 teaspoon of the mix in the bottom of the cup and pour the hot water over it.

4. Let it steep for 5 minutes, then strain and drink.

Consumption: Drink 1 cup of hot infusion every night before going to bed. You may consume it until the quality of your sleep has improved.

Mixed Infusion

Ingredients:

- 1 cup of water

- 1 oz of dried Willow

- 1 oz of dried Marjoram

- 1 oz of dried Lemon Balm

- 1 oz of dried Lavender

Preparation:

1. In a mason jar, mix all the herbs together.

2. Heat a cup of water well, without bringing it to a boil.

3. Put 1 teaspoon of the mix in the bottom of the cup and pour the hot water over it.

4. Let it steep for 5 minutes, then strain and drink.

Consumption: Drink 1 cup of hot infusion every night before going to bed. You may consume it until the quality of your sleep has improved.

Relaxing Infusion

Ingredients:

- 1 cup of water

- 1 oz of dried Damiana

- 1 oz of dried Oats

- 1 oz dried Alfalfa

Preparation:

1. In a mason jar, mix the herbs together.

2. Heat the water very well, without bringing it to a boil.

3. Put 1 teaspoon of mixture in the bottom of the cup and pour the hot water over it.

4. Let it steep for 10 minutes, then strain through a strainer.

Consumption: Drink 1 cup a day, preferably hot. It can be useful for relaxing before going to bed.

Slow Bowels and Constipation

Proper nutrition is most useful in relieving this disorder. In particular, foods such as grapes, plums, peaches, blackberries, apples, cherries, and oranges, are particularly useful, as far as fruits are concerned. For what concerns vegetables we have carrots, cooked green leafy vegetables, eggplant, onions, spinach, and tomatoes.

A very useful remedy in times of constipation is taking a tablespoon of extra-virgin olive oil every morning on an empty stomach, mixed with a teaspoon of freshly squeezed organic lemon juice. It is a remedy to be used for constipation days until the evacuation.

Chicory Infusion

Ingredients:

- 3 cups of water

- 0,7 oz of dried Chicory flowers

Preparation:

1. Heat the water well, without bringing it to a boil.

2. Put the Chicory in the bottom of the teapot and pour the hot water over it.

3. Let it steep for 10 minutes, then strain and place in a pitcher where you will keep it for the day.

Consumption: Drink 3 cups a day before each meal.

Mixed Infusion

Ingredients:

- 1 cup of water

- 0,35 oz of dried Licorice

- 0,15 oz of dried Fennel

- 0,15 oz of dried mallow

Preparation:

1. Heat the water well, without bringing it to a boil.

2. Put the herbs in the bottom of the cup and pour the hot water over them.

3. Let it steep for 7 minutes, then strain and drink.

Consumption: Drink 1 hot cup in the evening, after dinner.

Fig Decoction

Ingredients:

- 4 cups of water

- 4 or 5 dried Figs depending on size

Preparation:

1. Bring the water to a boil then add the dried Figs, after crushing them well.

2. Boil for 5 minutes over low heat and then strain well, crushing the pulp well to extract the liquid.

3. Pour it into a pitcher with a lid

Consumption: Drink the whole decoction throughout the day.

Sore Throat

Antiseptic Decoction

Ingredients:

- 4 cups of water

- 1,4 oz of dried Elderberries

- 0,2 oz of dried Ginger

- 3 Cloves

- 1 tablespoon honey

Preparation:

1. Bring water to a boil then add the herbs.

2. Simmer for 10 minutes and then strain.

3. Pour it into a jug with a stopper. Before closing the jug and before the decoction cools, add the honey and stir to dissolve it.

Consumption: Drink 3 cups throughout the day.

Basil Infusion

Ingredients:

- 4 cups of water

- 1,7 oz of dried Basil leaves

Preparation:

1. Heat the water very well, without bringing it to a boil.

2. Put the Basil in the bottom of the teapot and pour the hot water over it.

3. Let it steep for 10 minutes, then strain through a strainer.

4. Pour the infusion into a pitcher with a lid.

Use: Use the infusion to gargle 3 or 4 times daily for pain relief.

Stomachache

Soothing Infusion

Ingredients:

- 1 cup of water

- 0,7 oz of dried Chamomile

- 0,7 oz of dried Valerian

- 0,7 oz of dried Lemon Balm

Preparation:

1. In an airtight glass jar, mix the herbs together.

2. Heat the water very well, without bringing it to a boil.

3. Put 1 teaspoon of mixture in the bottom of the cup and pour the hot water over it.

4. Let it steep for 10 minutes, then strain through a strainer.

Consumption: Drink the infusion hot, but not boiling, when you need to soothe discomfort.

Stretch marks

Horsetail Decoction

Ingredients:

- 4 cups of water

- 1,8 oz dry stems of Horsetail

Preparation:

1. Bring the water to a boil then add the dried stems.

2. Boil for 10 minutes on low heat then strain.

3. Pour into a bowl and let it cool.

Use: Use the decoction to create tablets by soaking gauze or some cotton. Apply the decoction-soaked compresses directly to the stretch marks.

Toothache and Gums Ache

To decrease the pain of a toothache, the first step is to chew a mallow leaf. If the pain is caused by a cavity, you can insert a clove into the hole.

Herbal Macerate

Ingredients:

- 4 cups of 90° alcohol

- 0,7 oz of dried Thyme

- 0,7 oz of dried Oregano

- 0,7 oz of dried Rosemary

Preparation:

1. Place the alcohol and herbs in a covered container suitable for steeping. Put the container in a dark place or, at least, away from light sources.

2. Leave to macerate for 15 days, then strain very well using a strainer.

3. Transfer the macerate to a dark glass bottle that has a stopper to seal tightly and store the product.

Use: You will need to use the macerate whenever you have a toothache, rinsing and holding it in your mouth for at least 30 seconds, as you would with mouthwash.

Infusion for Inflamed Gums

Ingredients:

- 4 cups of water

- 1,7 oz of dried Mallow

Preparation:

1. Heat the water very well, without bringing it to a boil.

2. Put the Mallow in the bottom of a teapot and pour the hot water over it.

3. Let it steep for 15 minutes, then strain through a strainer.

4. Pour the infusion into a pitcher with a lid.

Consumption: Drink 2 or 3 cups throughout the day, away from meals.

Urticaria

Mixed Infusion

Ingredients:

- 3 cups water

- 0,5 oz of dried Meadowsweet

- 0,5 oz of dried Thyme

- 0,5 oz of dried Yarrow

- 0,2 oz of dried Mint

Preparation:

1. Heat the water very well, without bringing it to a boil.

2. Put the herbs in the bottom of a teapot and pour the hot water over them.

3. Let it steep for 5 minutes, then strain through a strainer.

4. Pour the infusion into a pitcher with a lid.

Consumption: Drink 3 cups a day after meals.

Mixed Infusion

Ingredients:

- 2 cups of water

- 0,35 oz of dried Rosemary

- 0,35 oz of dried Lemon Balm

- 0,2 oz of dried Gentian

Preparation:

1. Heat the water very well, without bringing it to a boil.

2. Put the herbs in the bottom of a teapot and pour the hot water over them.

3. Let it steep for 4 minutes, then strain through a strainer.

4. Pour the infusion into a pitcher with a lid.

Consumption: Drink 2 cups a day at your favorite time.

Wrinkles

Anti-Wrinkle Tablets

Ingredients:

- 4 cups of water

- 1,7 oz dried Rosemary (flowers and leaves)

Preparation:

1. Heat the water very well, without bringing it to a boil.

2. Put the Rosemary in the bottom of a teapot and pour the hot water over it.

3. Let it steep for 10 minutes, then strain through a strainer.

4. Put in a glass bottle with a stopper to store the infusion between uses.

Use: Using absorbent cotton pads, create compresses. Soak them well with the anti-wrinkle infusion and apply the compresses to the face and neck, every night before going to bed.

Wounds

In case of a superficial wound that is slow to heal, use:

Thyme Infusion

Ingredients:

- 1 cup of water

- 0,3 oz of dried Thyme

Preparation:

1. Heat the water well, without bringing it to a boil.

2. Put the leaves in the bottom of the cup and pour the hot water over them.

3. Let it steep for 30 minutes, then strain and place in a bowl.

Use: Make sure the infusion is well chilled before using. Dab the injured skin with gauze soaked in the infusion.

Holly Decoction

Ingredients:

- 1/2 cup of water

- 1.8 oz of dried Holly

Preparation:

1. Bring the water to a boil then add the holly.

2. Boil for 15-20 minutes (it should boil thoroughly, but not evaporate all the water).

3. Allow the decoction to cool.

Use: Apply Holly directly to injured skin. Holly has an astringent and hemostatic function and strengthens capillaries.

Yarrow Compress

Ingredients:

• Fresh Yarrow leaves, just enough

Preparation:

1. Finely chop fresh Yarrow leaves.

Use: Apply the chopped leaves directly to the injured skin. This use of yarrow is also good on sores.

TIP: You can also use an infusion of Yarrow, prepared with amounts and timing of that of thyme. The application also remains the same and has a hemostatic effect.

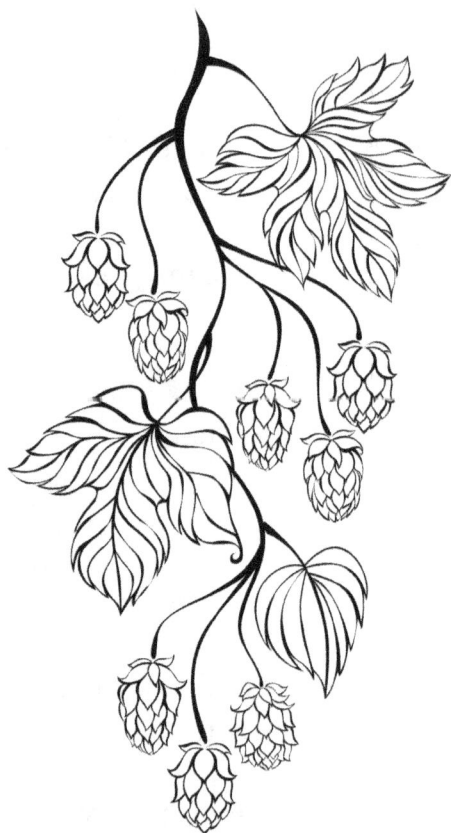

Hops

Conclusion

Here we are at the final chapter. I would like to thank you for sticking with me to the end, and I hope that you have enjoyed our time together as much as I have.

I will be happy if you would like to share your opinion with me, leaving a review or even just stars, to tell me what you think about this book.

I hope I was able to convey to you the importance of taking care of yourself and doing it in the most natural way possible. This way of taking care of myself by taking advantage of nature's resources has made a huge difference in the quality of my life, and I hope it will be the same for you. I wish you that this is the beginning of a journey that will make you feel better with each passing day. Drink your infusions and decoctions, eat more fruits and vegetables, make your own cosmetics, shampoos, and creams, and enjoy the benefits of nature's energy.

Remember that the purpose of this book is not to substitute traditional medicine cures for natural medicine cures. If you are suffering from any illness, your doctor is always the first person you should deal with.

Natural medicine and treating yourself with herbs and plants is additional support to traditional medicines and also a great way to take care of yourself daily, even and especially on a preventive level. Many of the remedies in this book also help you take care of all the little things you don't go and bother your doctors with, such as stretch marks, pimples, wrinkles, and such.

I divided the recipes in the book so it was easy to identify the use of certain plants and herbs with discomfort. What I do, is always keep a good supply of herbs with different properties and prepare decoctions and infusions throughout my day, according to the season, even before an uneasiness arises.

Instead of drinking chemical and carbonated drinks, I prepare delicious infusions and decoctions that I consume throughout my day, even during meals. I also carry them with me in my thermal water bottles so that I always have a healthy alternative with me. So make good use of all the information you have learned and use it to bring real benefit to your life.

It's been a tough couple of years for the health of us all, so take care of yourself and your body because it can only do you good. Taking care of yourself using plants means respecting your body's natural balance. In this way, you can prevent and relieve all those little discomforts that are caused in today's society by too hectic lifestyles, negative external stimuli, and constantly worsening eating habits.

I wish you a good life and hope our paths meet again in another one of my books or elsewhere.

NAMASTÉ

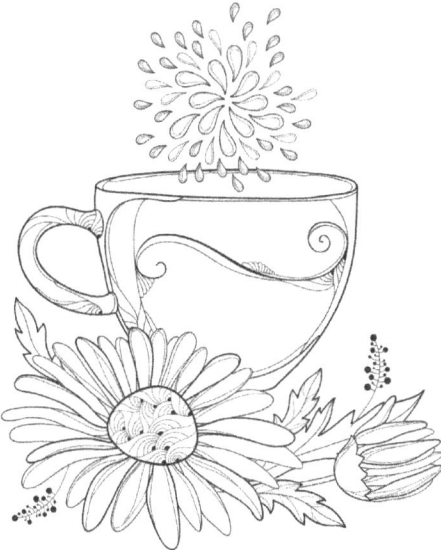

www.ingramcontent.com/pod-product-compliance
Lightning Source LLC
Chambersburg PA
CBHW020253030426
42336CB00010B/736